your guide to

lung
cancer

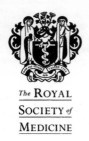

The ROYAL
SOCIETY of
MEDICINE

your guide to
lung
cancer

Dr David Gilligan
FRCP, FRCR
Dr Robert Rintoul
PhD, MRCP

Hodder Arnold
A MEMBER OF THE HODDER HEADLINE GROUP

Hodder Arnold have agreed to pay 50 pence per product on all sales made of this title to the retailer at a discount of up to and including 60% from the UK Recommended Retail Price to the British Lung Foundation.

Orders: Please contact Bookpoint Ltd, 130 Milton Park, Abingdon, Oxon OX14 4SB. Telephone: (44) 01235 827720, Fax: (44) 01235 400454. Lines are open from 9.00 to 18.00, Monday to Saturday, with a 24-hour message answering service. You can also order through our website www.hoddereducation.com.

British Library Cataloguing in Publication Data
A catalogue record for this title is available from the British Library.

ISBN-10: 0 340 927860
ISBN-13: 9 780340 927861

First published	2007			
Impression number	10 9 8 7 6 5 4 3 2 1			
Year	2010	2009	2008	2007

Typeset by Servis Filmsetting Limited, Longsight, Manchester.
Printed in Great Britain for Hodder Arnold, a division of Hodder Headline, 338 Euston Road, London NW1 3BH, by Cox & Wyman Ltd, Reading, Berkshire.

Hodder Headline's policy is to use papers that are natural, renewable and recyclable products and made from wood grown in sustainable forests. The logging and manufacturing processes are expected to conform to the environmental regulations of the country of origin.

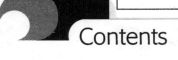

Contents

While every effort has been made to ensure that the
contents of this book are as accurate and up to date as
possible, neither the publishers nor the authors can be
held responsible for errors or for any consequences arising
from the use of information contained herein.

*Do not attempt to self-diagnose or self-treat for any
serious or long-term problems – always seek advice first
from a medical professional or qualified practitioner.*

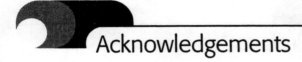

Acknowledgements

The authors and publishers would like to thank the following for their help with this book:

Gillian Stent, Susie Harden, Francis Wells, Mick Peake, Nick Screaton, Doris Rassl and Maureen King.

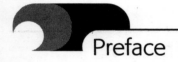

Preface

This new book, published in partnership with the Royal Society of Medicine, provides detailed, useful and up-to-date information on lung cancer. It contains expert yet user-friendly advice, with such useful features as:

Key Terms: demystifying the jargon
Questions and Answers: answering the burning questions
Myths and Facts: debunking the misconceptions
My Experience: how it feels to live with, or care for someone with, this condition.

Bearing the hallmark of excellence and accessibility that characterizes the work of the Royal Society of Medicine, this important guide will enable you and your family to gain some control over the way your lung cancer is managed by being better informed.

Peter Richardson
Director of Publications
Royal Society of Medicine

Introduction

Lung cancer is a common but often forgotten disease. It is the second most common cancer and is now almost as common in women as men. It has never had a high profile amongst cancers and one reason for this is that there is a strong association with cigarette smoking as the main cause for the disease. It is often perceived that people diagnosed with lung cancer have somehow inflicted the disease upon themselves. However, many people may have started smoking and become addicted to tobacco many years before the full health implications were known. Others may have struggled and succeeded in giving up years ago but are still at a higher risk of getting the disease. A significant minority of people will have never smoked.

One other reason is the perception that lung cancer is incurable, inevitably fatal, and that there are no effective treatments for the condition. This is not the case.

This book is designed to educate and provide information about lung cancer. It is aimed at those directly affected by lung cancer, either personally or through family or friends. It is also for those interested in finding out about this rarely publicized cancer. We have designed the book in such a way that the reader can either find out about the disease as a whole or dip into a particular aspect, for instance, how a diagnosis is made or a specific type of treatment.

Lung cancer can manifest itself in many ways and treatments can range from curative ones to those where the aim is to control the symptoms of advanced disease. It is important for all to realize that living with a cancer is possible. Achieving a good quality of life as well as quantity of life are goals for people with lung cancer and those involved in helping people with a diagnosis of lung cancer. Advances are taking place to improve care in every aspect of lung cancer through research and development. Most of these are not large changes but a number of small but definite steps which ultimately improve cure and control rates.

We hope that this book answers the questions you may have about lung cancer and also helps you in asking healthcare professionals further questions.

Dr David Gilligan
Dr Robert Rintoul

CHAPTER

1

Facts and figures

The lungs

Our lungs allow us to breathe. They are part of the respiratory system which is made up of the nose and mouth and the airways that lead down into the lungs (see Figure 1.1). The windpipe or **trachea** splits into two airways, one leading to each lung. These airways are called the right **main bronchus** and the left main bronchus. Within the lungs the bronchi split into smaller tubes called **lobar bronchi** which lead into the **lobes** of the lung. The right lung is divided into three lobes called the upper lobe, the middle lobe and the lower lobe (see Figure 1.2). The left lung has only two lobes, an upper and a lower. Within the lobes the lobar bronchi divide again and again into very fine breathing tubes

trachea
Air tube, usually stiffened by rings of cartilage, that extends from the voicebox to the bronchus of each lung.

main bronchus
An airway that supplies air to one lung.

lobar bronchi
A bronchus that supplies one lobe of the lung.

lobe
Segment of the lung.

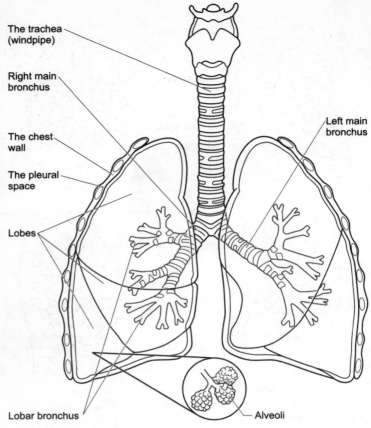

The trachea
(windpipe)

Right main
bronchus

The chest
wall

The pleural
space

Lobes

Left main
bronchus

Lobar bronchus

Alveoli

Figure 1.1 The basic structure of the lungs.

alveoli
The minute air sacs found at the end of the bronchial tubes. There are several million in each lung and it is through these that oxygen passes into the bloodstream and carbon dioxide passes out of the bloodstream.

pleura
Membrane lining the lung (visceral pleura) and the inside of the rib cage (parietal pleura).

which eventually end in millions of air sacs or **alveoli** (see Figure 1.1).

Each lung is covered by a membrane called the **pleura** (see Figure 1.3). Another similar membrane lines the inside of the rib cage. As we breathe the lungs inflate and deflate inside the chest. Normally there is a very small amount of fluid in the space between the two

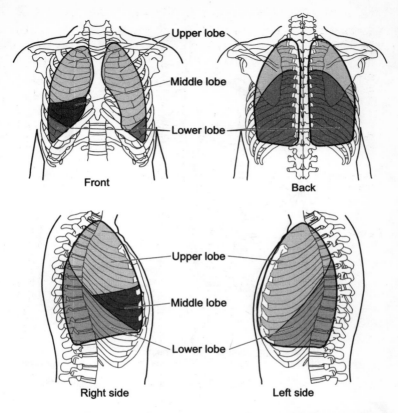

Front

Back

Right side

Left side

¶ Figure 1.2 The lobes of the lungs.

pleural membranes. This space is called the pleural space and the fluid, pleural fluid. The pleural fluid lubricates the pleural space so that the lungs move smoothly as they inflate and deflate. If too much fluid builds up in the pleural space, the lungs cannot expand as much as normal and you can become breathless. This is called a pleural effusion (see Figure 1.3).

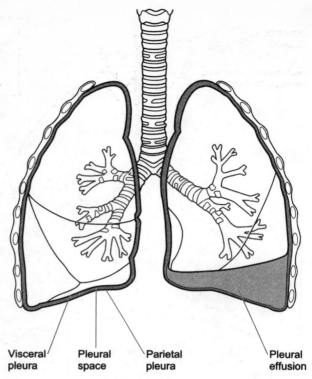

Visceral   Pleural   Parietal   Pleural
pleura   space   pleura   effusion

Figure 1.3 Pleural membranes of the lungs.

The lymph nodes

Lymph nodes or lymph glands are part of the lymphatic system which occurs throughout the body. Lymph nodes are small bean-shaped glands that are connected together by a fine system of vessels called **lymphatic vessels**. As blood circulates around the body, clear fluid leaks out of the blood vessels and bathes the cells with nutrients and oxygen. In turn, the cells pass out waste products and carbon dioxide. Some of the fluid passes directly back into the veins but the rest of the fluid is collected by the

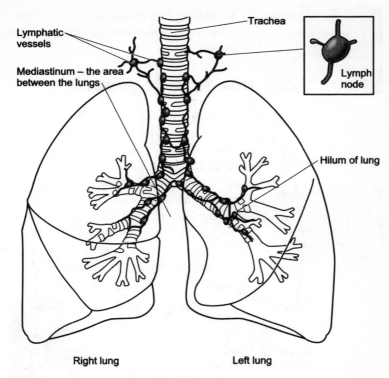

§ Figure 1.4 The lymph glands of the lungs.

lymph system and is filtered by the lymph glands. This fluid, called lymph fluid, is then passed back into the veins too. In cancer, the lymphatic system is very important because it is one of the ways that cancer cells can spread around the body. Therefore, in assessing how far a cancer has spread, cancer specialists are always keen to find out if any cancer cells have spread to the lymph glands. In the chest, there are lymph glands at the **hilum** of the lungs and around the large airways (main bronchi and the trachea) (see Figure 1.4). The area between the lungs in which the windpipe and main bronchi

hilum
The root of the lungs where the lobar bronchi join the main bronchi.

mediastinum
The area between the lungs that contains the heart, major blood vessels, gullet and windpipe.

lie is called the **mediastinum**. Lung cancers can also spread to the lymph glands at the base of the neck.

How do the lungs work?

The air that we breathe contains oxygen. The function of the lungs is to draw air into the body and then absorb the oxygen from the air into the bloodstream. The oxygen is then carried by the blood to every cell in the body. As we breathe in,

abdominal cavity
The cavity that holds the stomach, liver, gallbladder, spleen, pancreas, urinary bladder and intestines.

muscles in our chest cause the chest wall to move outwards and the diaphragm to move downwards. The diaphragm is a sheet of muscle that separates the chest cavity (above) from the **abdominal cavity** (below) . As a result of this

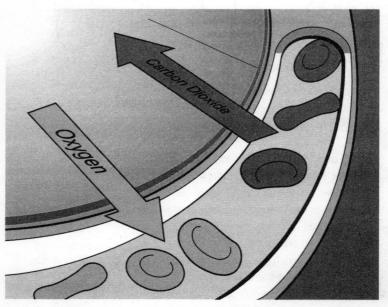

Figure 1.5 Oxygen and carbon dioxide gas exchange mechanism across the alveolar membrane.

Epidemiology of lung cancer

Lung cancer is the second most common cancer in the United Kingdom. Only breast cancer is more common. At present, there are 38,000 new cases of lung cancer each year in the UK. This represents about one in six new cases of cancer. Around nine out of ten people who develop lung cancer are, or have been, smokers. In the 1970s and 1980s the **incidence** of lung cancer in men in the UK was the highest in the world. Because of the poor survival rates from lung cancer the death rate tends to mirror the incidence rate. Therefore, the death rate from lung cancer in men at this time was the highest it has ever been. Over the last 30 years there has been a decline in the number of men who smoke in the UK and as a result the incidence of lung cancer and the death rates in men are now falling. However, in recent years the incidence of lung cancer in women in the UK has been increasing as more women take up smoking. Figure 1.7 shows how the incidence of lung cancer for men and women in the UK has changed over the last 30 years.

There is about a 15–20 year lag phase between a change in the **prevalence** of smoking and a change in the incidence of lung cancer. Although the number of men who smoked fell in the 1980s and 1990s, the number of women who smoked increased during that time and as a result we are now seeing more cases of lung cancer in women than in the past. At present it appears that the number of women who are taking up smoking is beginning to level off but it will be many years before we begin to see a fall in the incidence and death rate of lung cancer in women.

epidemiology
The study of patterns of disease.

incidence
The number of new cases of a disease occurring per year.

myth
Men who smoke are more likely to develop lung cancer than women.

fact
Women who smoke are just as likely to develop lung cancer as men.

prevalence
A measure of how common a condition or activity is, at any one time.

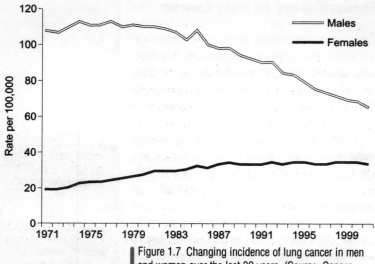

Figure 1.7 Changing incidence of lung cancer in men and women over the last 30 years. (Source: Cancer Starts Monograph 2004.)

risk factor
Anything that increases your chance of getting a disease.

myth
You cannot get lung cancer if you have never smoked.

fact
About one in ten people who get lung cancer have never smoked. Other risk factors include passive smoking, exposure to asbestos, radon gas and some other chemicals.

What are the risk factors for lung cancer?

Age

The risk of developing lung cancer increases with age. Lung cancer is uncommon below the age of 50 and three-quarters of cases occur over the age of 63. However, it can occur at any age after adolescence albeit in very small numbers.

Smoking

Tobacco smoking is known to cause the vast majority of the cases of lung cancer. About nine out of ten people who develop lung cancer are, or have been, smokers. The risk of someone developing lung cancer is related to how many cigarettes they smoke and how long they have movement air is drawn in through the nose and mouth and down into the lungs. Once the air reaches the alveoli at the end of the bronchi, oxygen is absorbed into the bloodstream (see Figure 1.5). Waste products from the cells such as carbon dioxide pass back into the alveoli from the bloodstream and is breathed out.

What is lung cancer?

Any abnormal growth of cells in the body is called a 'tumour'. Tumours can either be **benign** or **malignant**. The difference between benign and malignant tumours is whether they are able to **metastasize** or not. However large a benign tumour becomes, it will never spread to other parts of the body. Malignant tumours, on the other hand, will always have the potential to spread and it is these tumours that are called 'cancer'. Lung cancer is a malignant tumour which starts off in the lungs and although, initially, it may be limited to one lung, it will eventually spread to other parts of the body. The majority of lung cancers start in the cells lining the bronchi and are called carcinomas of the bronchus or bronchogenic carcinomas.

How does lung cancer develop?

There has been a lot of scientific research to try to find out how lung cancer develops and why some people get it and others don't. The most widely accepted theory is that it is a process involving many changes or **mutations** in the **genes** that control the way a cell grows and works. These mutations can cause activation of cancer promoting genes (**oncogenes**) or

benign
A non-cancerous tumour.

malignant
A tumour that is able to spread and grow in other parts of the body.

metastasize
The ability of a cancer to spread to other parts of the body to form secondary cancers (metastases). Lung cancers commonly spread to the liver, brain, bones, other lung and adrenal glands in the abdomen.

mutation
Alteration in the DNA sequence of a cell.

gene
Sequence of DNA required to produce a protein.

oncogene
Tumour gene present in the body that can be activated and cause cells to grow and divide in an uncontrolled manner.

Q **Both my parents were smokers and died of lung cancer. Will I get it too?**

A There is some evidence that the children or siblings of people with lung cancer are more likely to develop it if they also smoke. However, at present there is no scientific way of predicting who is going to develop lung cancer and who is not. The best thing you can do is not to smoke at all. If you do not smoke the chance of developing lung cancer is very small whatever your family history.

switching off of cancer protecting genes. Several mutations in different genes may be required to turn a normal cell into a cancerous cell. At first the changes to a cell may be reversible but as more and more mutations occur the changes become irreversible and a cancerous cell develops (see Figure 1.6). It is now realized that the many **carcinogens** in cigarette smoke can cause the genetic changes required to turn a normal cell into a cancer cell. However, if this is the case, why doesn't everyone who smokes get lung cancer? The answer to this question is not fully understood yet but it is possible that the types of genes you inherit may partly determine your risk of lung cancer. If these people also smoke they may be more likely to get lung cancer. At present this remains a scientific theory as no major genes for lung cancer have been identified as yet.

carcinogen
A cancer promoting agent.

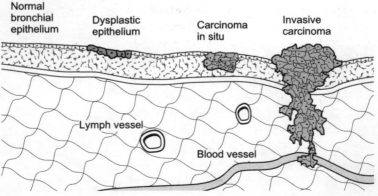

Normal bronchial epithelium   Dysplastic epithelium   Carcinoma in situ   Invasive carcinoma

Lymph vessel

Blood vessel

Figure 1.6 Stages of lung cancer development.

been smoking. Compared with someone who has never smoked, a person who smokes between one and 14 cigarettes per day has eight times more risk of dying from lung cancer. Someone who smokes 25 cigarettes per day is 25 times more likely to die from lung cancer than someone who has never smoked. However, the length of time someone has been smoking is more important than how many cigarettes they smoke.

We now know that if you have smoked 20 a day for 40 years, your risk of lung cancer is about eight times greater than if you smoked 40 a day for 20 years. However, if someone who has been smoking for many years stops, they can avoid much of their subsequent risk of lung cancer (see Figure 1.8). Following permanent smoking cessation the risk of developing lung cancer falls

myth
Smoking low tar cigarettes decreases the chance of developing lung cancer.

fact
There is no evidence that if you smoke low tar cigarettes you are less likely to develop lung cancer.

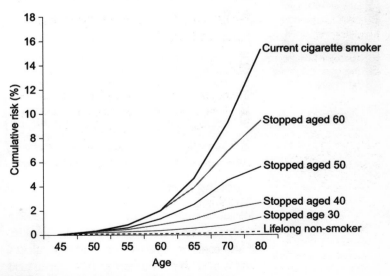

Figure 1.8 Effects of stopping smoking at various ages on the cumulative risk (%) of death from lung cancer by age 75 for men in the UK. (Source: Cancer Research UK.)

myth

Smoking a pipe does not cause lung cancer.

fact

Smoking a pipe and smoking cigars are risk factors for lung cancer. Pipe smokers are also more at risk of cancers of the lips and mouth.

Q I work in a smoky environment. Am I at risk of lung cancer?

A Research has shown that people who are regularly exposed to cigarette smoke in the workplace are about 20 per cent more likely to get lung cancer than someone who does not work in a smoky atmosphere.

rapidly. After 15 to 20 years as a non-smoker the risk of developing lung cancer will drop to only about twice that of someone who has never smoked. Thus stopping smoking at almost any age will have a significant impact on the risk of an individual developing lung cancer.

Passive smoking

In the last few years there has been a lot of concern about the risk of passive smoking which is also known as 'second-hand' smoke i.e. breathing in the cigarette smoke from someone else's cigarette. It is now recognized that passive smoking can cause lung cancer. A non-smoker who is married to a smoker has up to a 30 per cent greater risk of developing lung cancer compared to someone who is married to a non-smoker.

my experience

When I became breathless recently, I went to see my GP who organized a chest X-ray. This showed a shadow and I have now been diagnosed with lung cancer. I was very shocked when I heard the diagnosis because I have never smoked. However, the doctors believe that I have probably developed it as a result of passive smoking or 'second hand' smoke. I run a pub and have spent many years working in a very smoky atmosphere.

Smoking marijuana

Marijuana contains many of the cancer-causing compounds that are found in ordinary cigarettes. It also contains more tar than ordinary cigarettes and is often inhaled deeply and the smoke held in the lungs for longer than ordinary cigarettes. Smoking marijuana is thought to be a risk factor for lung cancer but it is difficult to carry out research on it as it is illegal to smoke and many people do not admit to smoking it. Also many marijuana smokers are also cigarette smokers so it is difficult to separate the risks of smoking marijuana from the risks associated with smoking cigarettes.

Asbestos

Exposure to asbestos is a risk factor for lung cancer as well as being a risk factor for **asbestos related lung disease**. Death from lung cancer among people who have been exposed to asbestos is about seven times more common than among the general population. However, if people who have been previously exposed to asbestos also smoke, the risk of developing lung cancer is many times higher. Some estimates put it as high as 50 times greater than among the general population. Therefore, it is essential for people who have been exposed to asbestos in the past to stop smoking.

asbestos related lung disease
Asbestos can cause a number of conditions that affect the lung or the lining of the lung including benign pleural plaques, asbestosis and malignant mesothelioma.

Radon gas

Radon is a naturally occurring radioactive gas produced by the breakdown of uranium. A link between radon and lung cancer was first identified in uranium miners who were exposed to high levels of radon. Normally radon does not pose any threat to us as it is present in such tiny amounts but, in some parts of the UK such as the West Country and the north of Scotland where there is a lot of granite in the soil, it has been found that it can build up inside buildings to high levels. It is thought that radon gas in high concentrations may cause lung cancer.

Exposure to chemicals

Exposure to certain carcinogen-containing chemicals such as uranium, nickel, arsenic, zinc, polycyclic hydrocarbons and chromium are believed to be able to cause lung cancer. This risk appears to be independent of smoking. However, very few people work with such chemicals and nowadays the regulations in the UK are very strict so there should be very few cases due to these causes in the future.

Air pollution and diesel fumes

It is believed that heavy exposure to diesel fumes probably increases the risk of developing lung cancer and outdoor air pollution in built-up areas may also make a small contribution to the risk of developing the disease. However, because these risks are very low they are very difficult to study and separate from other risks such as smoking.

Family history of lung cancer

If you have had lung cancer in the past you are at a higher risk of developing another lung cancer. There is also now some evidence that the brothers, sisters and children of those who have had lung cancer may be at a slightly higher risk of developing lung cancer themselves, especially if they smoke too. At present there is a considerable amount of research being undertaken to look at these risks and to try to determine if risk can be inherited in the genes. However, to date, no specific gene has been associated with lung cancer.

my experience

Although I have never smoked I am concerned that I might develop lung cancer. My brother, father and uncle have all had lung cancer although unlike me they were all smokers. I have talked to my GP about this and he explained that it is thought that there may be genes in some families that put them at a higher risk of developing lung cancer but that at present there are no tests available to find out what my particular risk is. However, the fact that I have never smoked is a good thing. I feel that it is very important that my children know about our family history so they understand why they should never smoke.

Previous cancer treatment

There is some evidence that people who have had previous radiotherapy to their chest or for **Hodgkin's disease** may be at increased risk of lung cancer, especially if they smoke. However, the risk is reduced with modern radiotherapy techniques and lower doses of radiotherapy.

Hodgkin's disease
A type of lymphoma – cancer of the lymph glands.

Scarring from previous lung disease

It is thought that some people who have scarring within their lungs from other causes may be at an increased risk of lung cancer. Some lung cancers appear to start off in areas of old lung scarring. Patients with **lung fibrosis** seem to be particularly prone to developing lung cancer especially if they also smoke.

lung fibrosis
Lung fibrosis involves scarring of the lung. Gradually, the air sacs of the lungs become replaced by fibrotic tissue. When the scar forms, the tissue becomes thicker causing an irreversible loss of the tissue's ability to transfer oxygen into the bloodstream. In some cases no cause can be identified – this is called idiopathic lung fibrosis.

Screening programmes for lung cancer

Screening programmes for cancers such as breast cancer and cervical cancer are already well developed and widely practised. At present there is no routine lung cancer screening programme in the UK. There have previously been attempts to improve the survival of smokers by screening for lung cancer using regular chest X-rays to detect small cancers before they cause symptoms. However, these attempts were not successful in reducing lung cancer death rates. Currently there are a number of experimental clinical trials being undertaken in various countries using annual **CT scans** to try to find out whether this is a good method of reducing death rates from lung cancer. Another approach that is undergoing scientific testing is autofluorescence bronchoscopy. During a bronchoscopy test (see Chapter 3 for details) a special blue light is shone on the inside of the airways in order to highlight abnormal areas which may be in the process of becoming cancerous. Although promising, the results of these trials will not be available for several years.

CT scan
Computed tomography scan.

Types of lung cancer

Cancer affecting the lung can either be due to cancer that has started in the lung (primary lung cancer) or cancer that has spread to the lung from somewhere else (secondary lung cancer). When a doctor says that someone has lung cancer they are usually talking about primary lung cancer. This book deals mainly with primary lung cancer.

Primary lung cancer is split into two groups:

✧ non-small cell lung cancer (NSCLC)
✧ small cell lung cancer (SCLC).

Non-small cell lung cancer accounts for about 80 per cent of cases of lung cancer and small cell lung cancer for the remaining 20 per cent. Doctors separate lung cancer into these two groups because experience has shown that they usually behave differently and respond to treatment differently.

Non-small cell lung cancer

Non-small cell lung cancer is usually divided into three different types depending on its appearance under the microscope. The three types are:

✧ squamous cell carcinoma
✧ adenocarcinoma
✧ large cell carcinoma.

Squamous cell carcinoma

Squamous cell carcinoma is the most common type of non-small cell carcinoma seen in the UK. It accounts for about 40 per cent of cases of lung cancer at present; although in the last few years the number of cases of this type has been falling in some countries. In North America the proportion of squamous cell carcinomas has fallen from 40 per cent to 20–25 per cent. Squamous cell lung cancer is usually due to smoking and it usually starts in the cells that line the major airways (bronchi). As a result it is often seen near the centre of the lungs in one of the main bronchi. Squamous cell carcinoma tends to grow more slowly than the other types of lung cancer and spreads at a later stage.

Adenocarcinoma

Adenocarcinoma is thought to develop from glandular cells located in the lining of the airways.

Adenocarcinomas often arise in the outer part of the lung but can sometimes spread to the lymph glands or to other parts of the body at an early stage. Adenocarcinomas account for about 25 per cent of all cases of lung cancer in the UK. However, in some countries such as North America it is becoming more common and is now more prevalent than squamous cell lung cancer. Some specialists believe that this change may be related to more women taking up smoking, as this type is more common in women. Adenocarcinoma is also the most common type of lung cancer to occur in people who have never smoked.

Among people who get adenocarcinoma, some develop a particular type called bronchoalveolar cell carcinoma. Bronchoalveolar cell carcinoma usually arises towards the edge of the lung in the alveoli. In general, these tumours grow fairly slowly and may cause few symptoms at first, which allows them to get quite large before they are detected. Sometimes they can occur in several places in one lung or in both lungs. Occasionally these tumours produce large amounts of mucus which results in patients coughing up large amounts of sputum, a symptom called bronchorrhoea.

Large cell carcinoma

Large cell carcinoma is a type of non-small cell lung cancer that lacks the specific features of adenocarcinoma or squamous cell carcinoma. It accounts for about ten per cent of all lung cancers. Large cell tumours are usually found in smokers and most of these tumours arise towards the edge of the lungs.

Q **Does it make a difference which type of non-small cell lung cancer I have?**

A At present all non-small cell lung cancers are treated in similar ways. The actual type of treatment offered depends more on the degree of spread or stage (see later in this chapter) rather than the particular type of cell. In fact, sometimes lung cancers may be made up of a mixture of more than one type of cell. Sometimes it is not possible for the pathologist to identify exactly which type of non-small cell lung cancer it is. In these cases they call it undifferentiated or poorly differentiated non-small cell lung cancer. Therefore, the actual type is less important. However, this may change in the future as new treatments are discovered. There is some evidence now that some drug treatments may be better for some types of non-small cell lung cancers than others. More detail about this is given in Chapter 6.

Small cell lung cancer

About one in five cases of lung cancer are due to small cell lung cancer. Small cell lung cancer gets its name because the cells appear small under the microscope and are largely filled by the **nucleus**. It used to be called 'oat cell' cancer because the cells were thought to resemble oat grains but this name is rarely used now. Almost all small cell lung cancer is caused by smoking – it is rare for someone who has never smoked, or been exposed to cigarette smoke, to develop it. Unfortunately, it is an aggressive type of lung cancer and in the majority of cases it has already spread to the lymph glands or to other parts of the body by the time it is discovered. Therefore, whenever possible lung cancer specialists advise treatment with chemotherapy. More detail about treatment for small cell lung cancer is given in Chapters 5 and 6. Occasionally (less than one per

nucleus
The control centre of a cell.

cent of cases) a very early small cell lung cancer is discovered and, if tests show that it has not spread to the lymph glands or to other parts of the body, surgery may be recommended, but this is unusual.

Secondary lung cancer

Several different types of cancer can spread to the lungs. Common types that do this are breast cancer, bowel cancer and kidney cancer. If a breast cancer spreads to the lungs the cells that do so are breast cancer cells, not lung cancer cells. Therefore, you will be treated for breast cancer not lung cancer. It is very important if you have had a cancer in the past to tell your specialist so that they can find out whether the cancer in the lung is actually a new primary lung cancer or whether it is your previous cancer which has come back and spread to the lungs. The treatment for another type of cancer which has spread to the lungs may be very different from that for primary lung cancer.

Other types of lung tumour

Hamartoma

Hamartomas are the most common type of benign (non-cancerous) lung tumour. They are formed from lung tissue that has developed in an unusual or disorganized fashion. They are usually quite small but can grow up to five centimetres in size. Most cause no symptoms at all but sometimes they can cause symptoms such as a cough or lung infections, especially if they are growing in an airway. They are sometimes found by chance when a chest X-ray or CT scan is done for some other reason. Sometimes they can be confidently diagnosed by scans or by performing a biopsy. In these cases no further treatment is needed. Occasionally, however, if they are causing symptoms or if a biopsy has not given a clear diagnosis, surgical removal is recommended. Hamartomas never become cancerous or re-occur following removal.

Carcinoid tumours

Carcinoid tumours are a rare form of tumour that can occur in various parts of the body including the lung. They belong to the family of **neuroendocrine tumours**. Carcinoid tumours are divided into typical carcinoids and atypical carcinoids depending upon their appearance under the microscope. The symptoms that they cause tend to depend on their location within the lung. Some develop in the walls of large airways near the centre of the lungs and others develop in the narrower airways towards the edges (periphery) of the lungs. Central carcinoid tumours can cause symptoms such as a cough, wheezing and coughing up of blood. If a large tumour blocks an airway it may cause symptoms of breathlessness or infection. Peripheral carcinoids may cause no symptoms at all and are sometimes detected by a chest X-ray or CT scan performed for some other purpose.

Occasionally, if the tumour spreads to the liver, it can cause a particular set of symptoms due to the release of hormone-like substances into the bloodstream. These symptoms are called **carcinoid syndrome** but they are rarely associated with lung carcinoids. The treatment of carcinoid tumours is beyond the scope of this

neuroendocrine tumours
There are several types of neuroendocrine lung tumours which arise from specialized cells in the lung called neuroendocrine cells. The most serious type is small cell lung cancer which is described earlier in this chapter. The other two main types of neuroendocrine tumours are typical and atypical carcinoids.

carcinoid syndrome
The symptoms of carcinoid syndrome commonly include flushing, diarrhoea, abdominal pain and wheezing.

book but in general, as long as the tumour has not spread to the liver, lung carcinoids can often be removed by surgery.

In addition to the tumours described here there are several other rare types of lung tumour. These affect a small number of people each year. Discussion of these is beyond the scope of this book.

Staging of lung cancer

Once a lung cancer has been diagnosed it is very important for the specialists to find out exactly which part of the lung it is lying in, how big it is, and whether it has spread. The answers to these questions will allow the doctors to work out which stage the cancer is at. This is important for deciding upon the most appropriate treatment. Following the diagnosis various tests often need to be performed in order to work out the stage the cancer has reached. More information about the different types of tests is given in Chapter 3.

The staging systems used for non-small cell lung cancer and small cell lung cancer are different.

Staging of non-small cell lung cancer

Doctors use an international classification system for many types of non-small cell lung cancer called the TNM system. This stands for tumour (T), lymph nodes (N) and metastases (M). The reason for performing tests to stage a lung cancer is to allow it to be classified using the TNM system.

The size and position of the primary lung cancer affects the T classification.

T1 Primary tumour less than 3 cm in diameter.

T2 Primary tumour more than 3 cm in diameter;

or

the tumour has grown into a main bronchus but lies more than 2 cm from the trachea;

or

the tumour has grown into the pleural membrane covering the lung;

or

the tumour has caused one of the lobes of the lung to collapse.

T3 The tumour has grown into a main bronchus and lies less than 2 cm from the trachea;

or

the tumour has grown into the chest wall or the diaphragm or the pericardium;

or

the tumour has grown into the pleural membrane separating the lung from the mediastinum (the mediastinal pleura);

or

the tumour has caused the whole lung to collapse.

T4 The tumour is growing into the structures in the mediastinum;

or

there is a pleural effusion present (fluid in the pleural space) which has been shown to contain cancer cells;

or

there is evidence that the tumour has spread to other parts of the same lobe of the lung that it started in.

Spread of cancer to lymph glands in the chest determines the N classification.

N0   No evidence of cancer in any lymph glands.

N1   Evidence of cancer in lymph glands at the root (hilum) of the lung.

N2   Evidence of cancer in lymph glands in the mediastinum on the same side as the primary tumour.

N3   Evidence of cancer in lymph glands in the mediastinum but on the opposite side to the primary tumour;
or
evidence of cancer in lymph glands that lie at the top of the lung around the collar bone (clavicle).

metastasis
The spread of a cancer from one part of the body to another via the bloodstream or lymphatic system.

Evidence of **metastasis** determines the M classification.

M0   No evidence of any spread to other lobes of the lung or to other parts of the body.

M1   There is evidence that the cancer has spread to another lobe of the same lung in which it started or to another part of the body.

In order to help guide treatment, lung cancer specialists group the TNM classes into stages which are numbered 1 to 4. Stage 1 contains tumours which are at the earliest stage of development and Stage 4 contains tumours which are at the most advanced stage.

Stage 1

This is divided into two sub-groups 1A and 1B.

Stage 1A   T1N0M0
Stage 1B   T2N0M0

Stage 2

This is divided into two sub-groups 2A and 2B.

Stage 2A   T1N1M0
Stage 2B   T2N1M0 or T3N0M0

Stage 3

This is divided into two sub-groups 3A and 3B.

Stage 3A   T1N2M0, T2N2M0, T3N1M0 or
            T3N2M0
Stage 3B   Any T, N3 M0 or T4, any N, M0

Stage 4

            Any T, Any N, M1

Staging of small cell lung cancer

Small cell lung cancer is divided into two stages:

✧ limited stage
✧ extensive stage.

Limited stage

About 30 per cent of new cases are diagnosed as limited stage. This means that the disease is limited to one lung and lymph glands in the centre of the chest or the root of the neck.

Extensive stage

Most new cases of small cell lung cancer are extensive stage at the time of diagnosis. This means that the cancer has spread beyond the lung that it started in to more distant lymph glands or to other organs in the body such as the liver or the brain.

Outcomes from lung cancer

prognosis
Forecast of the probable or expected outcome of a disease.

Several different factors influence a person's outcome or **prognosis** from lung cancer. These include the type of lung cancer, the patient's overall health, and the stage of the cancer at the time of diagnosis. All of these factors will influence the treatment that can be offered to a patient and this plays a large part in determining prognosis.

The type of lung cancer

The prognosis from small cell lung cancer is rather different from non-small cell lung cancer and therefore they are normally considered separately.

Overall health at the time of diagnosis

performance status
A simple 0–4 scale that describes everyday activities that a patient with cancer is capable of undertaking and their ability to have treatment.

The overall health of a patient at the time of diagnosis of lung cancer is important as it will influence the type of treatment that can be offered. This is called **performance status** (see Figure 1.9).

It is quite common for patients with lung cancer to have symptoms such as tiredness or weight loss which limits them in their day-to-day activities. These symptoms may also affect the type of treatment that can be offered and this in

Description	Score
Fully active	0
Restricted in strenuous activity, able to carry out light tasks	1
Capable of caring for self, up and about over 50 per cent of waking hours	2
Capable of limited self care, in bed or chair more than 50 per cent of waking hours	3
Totally confined to bed or chair, unable to look after self	4

Figure 1.9 Classification system for performance status (Eastern co-operative oncology group – ECOG).

turn may affect outcome. More details about performance status and how it can affect treatment are given in Chapter 6.

Closely linked to performance status are the effects that any other **co-morbidities** may have on the health of a patient. For instance, it is quite common for patients with lung cancer to also have chronic bronchitis and emphysema or heart disease. These conditions and many others may affect the type of treatment that can be offered.

> **co-morbidities**
> Other illnesses or conditions that a patient with lung cancer might have.

Stage of lung cancer

Prognosis from either type of lung cancer is related to the stage of the disease at the time of diagnosis. The earlier the stage of the cancer when it is first diagnosed the better the outcome.

Five-year survival

Cancer statistics often use the term 'five-year survival'. This refers to the percentage of people alive five years after a diagnosis of cancer. It is useful because it gives a way of comparing responses to different treatments for the various stages of cancer. However, although this is a useful way for a statistician to look at survival, it is very important to remember that the figures quoted are averages obtained from looking at what has happened to a large number of people with lung cancer of a similar stage. They cannot predict exactly what will happen to any one person. Survival at five years is used because, in general, if someone survives for five years after a diagnosis of cancer they are thought to be cured. However, although this is generally true for lung cancer it can sometimes come back more than five years later.

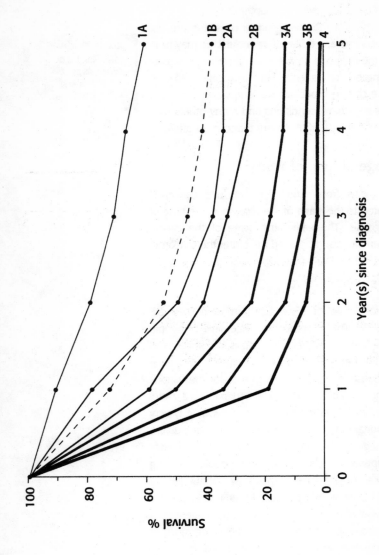

● Figure 1.10 Five-year survival according to stage of non-small cell lung cancer. For definitions of each stage see pages 24–5.

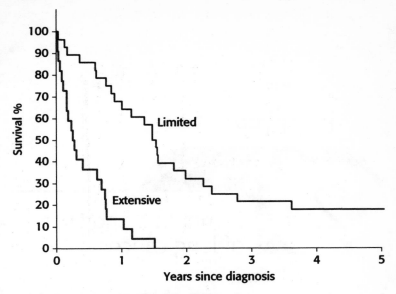

Figure 1.11 Five-year survival according to stage of small cell lung cancer.

Figure 1.10 shows the five-year survival curves for each stage of non-small cell lung cancer while Figure 1.11 shows the five-year survival for limited and extensive stage small cell lung cancer.

CHAPTER

2

Symptoms and signs of lung cancer

Most people with lung cancer will have some symptoms although sometimes, especially in the early stages, lung cancer may cause no symptoms at all. Some lung cancers are detected by chance when a patient has a chest X-ray or CT scan for some other reason. Although lung cancer can cause many different symptoms there are no symptoms which occur only in lung cancer. Many of the symptoms caused by lung cancer are quite common among the general population and as a result are sometimes ignored initially by the patient. This can result in a delay between the symptom first occurring and the patient going to their general practitioner (GP). A delay may result in the cancer becoming more advanced and more difficult to treat. Therefore, it is very important that patients report symptoms to their GP as soon as possible.

Initially the GP will take a history from the patient and perform a general examination. Depending upon the symptoms and signs, the GP may either refer the patient to a **consultant respiratory physician** immediately or treat symptoms to see if they go away. This is because many symptoms which could be due to lung cancer are often caused by less serious conditions and if GPs referred all patients to a specialist the system would be overwhelmed and those patients who really did need an urgent appointment would not be able to get one. A GP may arrange for a chest X-ray to be performed as this can often be helpful in determining whether a patient should be referred to a specialist urgently or whether it is appropriate to wait and see if symptoms get better by themselves or with some treatment such as antibiotics. Most patients who have symptoms with lung cancer will have an abnormal chest X-ray, but a normal chest X-ray does not completely rule out the diagnosis. Therefore, a GP may still refer such a patient to a specialist if he or she continues to have cause for concern.

> **consultant respiratory physician**
> A hospital-based doctor who specializes in lung diseases. Sometimes referred to as a chest physician or lung specialist.

Common symptoms

Some of the most common symptoms that can occur in lung cancer include:

Cough

Most people who develop lung cancer are, or have been, cigarette smokers and a cough is a common symptom in such people. However, a new cough or a change in an existing cough is a worrying symptom which should be reported to a doctor. Lung cancer can cause a cough because it irritates the inside of the airway. A cough is the most commonly reported symptom in patients presenting with lung cancer. If an unexplained cough is present for more than three weeks, a chest X-ray should be performed.

> **my experience**
>
> I had had a cough in the early morning for years which I had put down to my smoking. However, one day I noticed that recently my cough had changed and that I was coughing throughout the day. I mentioned this to my GP the next time I saw him and he suggested I have a chest X-ray. I am very glad that I did speak to my GP as the X-ray showed that I had an early stage of lung cancer.

Being short of breath

chronic bronchitis
Chronic inflammation of the airways caused by cigarette smoke.

emphysema
Irreversible destruction of lung tissue caused by cigarette smoke.

pleural effusion
Fluid that accumulates between the pleural membranes.

Smokers and ex-smokers often develop shortness of breath because of smoking-related **chronic bronchitis** and **emphysema**. However, worsening shortness of breath is concerning and should be reported to a doctor. It is likely that a chest X-ray will be arranged initially. Lung cancer can cause shortness of breath for several reasons. Sometimes a tumour can block or partly block one of the bronchi which can lead to collapse and infection in part of the lung. Lung cancers which affect the lining of the lung can cause fluid to build up around the lung. This is called a **pleural effusion** (see Figure 1.3 in Chapter 1). If a large amount of fluid builds up it can compress the lung which can cause breathlessness. Shortness of breath is the second most common symptom that patients with lung cancer report.

Coughing up blood

haemoptysis
A condition where the patient coughs up blood or sputum containing blood.

Coughing up blood or phlegm (sputum) that contains blood is a worrying symptom and will prompt most people to see their doctor. The medical term for this is **haemoptysis**. Although the majority of people who cough up blood will not have lung cancer, it is a common symptom of lung cancer and therefore anyone who coughs up blood should see their doctor immediately who will likely arrange a chest X-ray.

Repeated chest infections that are slow to clear up

Sometimes lung cancer can present as a chest infection which is slow to clear up or re-occurs after a short time. Patients, especially smokers or ex-smokers, who have been treated for a chest infection will often have a chest X-ray arranged in order to check that the infection has completely cleared up. If the chest X-ray is abnormal or if symptoms persist it is likely that their GP will refer them to a consultant respiratory physician for further investigations.

Tiredness

Tiredness or fatigue is a very common symptom which can be due to many different causes. However, unexplained symptoms in a smoker or ex-smoker need to be taken seriously and among the tests that a GP may do is a chest X-ray. If this shows anything abnormal or if other tests or examination findings give cause for concern it is likely that a referral to a specialist will result.

Noisy breathing

The most common type of 'noisy breathing' is a **wheeze** which is often heard in patients with asthma or chronic bronchitis. As with many

myth
Coughing up blood is always due to lung cancer.

fact
There are many reasons why people cough up blood. Although it can be due to lung cancer, the most common reason is a chest infection. However, it should always be taken seriously and anyone who coughs up blood should see their GP quickly. The GP will try and find out why it has happened and will start treatment if necessary.

wheeze
Audible, high-pitched musical noises usually heard when breathing out.

symptoms of lung cancer, a new wheeze in a person who smokes or has previously done so does not necessarily mean lung cancer but it should be reported to your doctor for further assessment.

Occasionally a lung cancer can cause narrowing of one of the main airways or the windpipe. This can cause a particular type of noise when breathing in called '**stridor**'. This is a serious symptom which should be investigated by a lung specialist urgently.

stridor
A high pitched, harsh noise caused by partial airway obstruction.

Q I have had a hoarse voice for several weeks now. I think it is due to smoking. Should I see my GP about it?

A Yes. Although it may be due to an infection, there is an increased risk of throat cancer and lung cancer in smokers and ex-smokers. Both can cause a persistent hoarse voice. Sometimes if a lung cancer develops at the top of the left lung it can damage a nerve that supplies the voice box. This can prevent one of the vocal cords from working properly, which can lead to a hoarse voice. Your GP will be able to arrange a chest X-ray and a referral to an ear, nose and throat specialist or a chest physician.

Losing weight unintentionally

Unexpected weight loss is a worrying symptom that will usually make a patient consult their doctor quickly. Although it can be due to many different causes it always needs to be investigated and, as part of those tests, the doctor will often request a chest X-ray or a CT scan. Weight loss of up to one stone (six kilograms) occurs in more than half of patients with lung cancer.

Developing a hoarse voice

A hoarse voice is a common symptom in the general population especially in those with head colds and chest infections. However, a hoarse voice in a smoker or ex-smoker that does not improve within two to three weeks should be investigated by a G.P.

New aches or pains in the chest or shoulders

Aches and pains in the chest or shoulders are commonly reported by patients with lung cancer, although they can also be due to muscular or heart problems. Persistent or worsening chest pain can be due to a lung cancer growing into the chest wall from the lung or due to a tumour in the ribs or spine. Sometimes lung cancer can develop at the top of the lungs (**Pancoast tumour**) and when it does it can cause shoulder pain which quite commonly can be mistaken for a frozen shoulder. This can sometimes lead to delay before the correct diagnosis is made. A chest X-ray taken when the symptoms first develop can often speed up the correct diagnosis. If a Pancoast tumour develops at the top of one lung it can sometimes cause a specific set of symptoms including drooping of the eyelid on that side, a small pupil in that eye and loss of sweating over the same side of the face. This group of symptoms is called Horner's syndrome and is due to the tumour causing damage to a nerve that runs up from the neck to supply the face.

Pancoast tumour
A lung cancer that develops, at the apex of the lung and invades nearby tissues such as the ribs and vertebrae.

Less common symptoms

In addition to the symptoms already listed, there are several less common symptoms which can be caused by lung cancer.

Superior vena cava obstruction (SVCO)

Superior vena cava obstruction or superior vena cava syndrome occurs if the superior vena cava becomes blocked. The superior vena cava is the main blood vessel that carries blood from the head and arms back to the heart. If it becomes blocked, blood backlogs in the head and arms resulting in swelling of the arms and face. This can cause headaches and an uncomfortable feeling of fullness in the face. Quite commonly, in its early stages, the symptoms of facial swelling can be mistaken for an allergic reaction.

Paraneoplastic syndromes

Some types of lung cancer can produce hormones and chemicals that can cause a variety of symptoms that people do not normally associate with lung cancer. These signs and symptoms are called paraneoplastic syndromes. The most common one of these symptoms is mild muscle weakness which can occur in ten to 20 per cent of patients with lung cancer. A variety of other neurological symptoms can occur but these are rare and tend to affect less than one per cent of people with lung cancer. They are more commonly seen in patients with small cell lung cancer. The production of hormones by some lung cancers can cause an imbalance of the salts in the blood and this can cause a variety of symptoms including weakness, dizziness and confusion.

Presenting symptoms caused by metastatic spread

Sometimes patients with lung cancer do not have any symptoms at all from the cancer in the lung but present with symptoms caused by metastatic spread of the cancer. Lung cancer most commonly spreads to the lymph glands, bones, liver and brain.

Lung cancer often spreads to lymph glands causing them to swell up and feel hard. The most common place that a patient might notice swollen lymph glands is in the side of the neck or just above the collar bones.

Bone metastases usually cause pain although sometimes they can cause a bone to break. The commonest bones affected are the spine, pelvis, ribs and the long bones of the arms and legs. Occasionally lung cancer presents with back pain due to a bone metastasis in the spine which is the cause of this pain. Sometimes the metastasis can put pressure on the spinal cord that lies within the spine and this can cause neurological symptoms in the arms or more commonly the legs such as weakness, numbness or pins and needles. This is an emergency called 'spinal cord compression' which requires urgent treatment with drugs and radiotherapy.

Liver metastases are often symptomless but can occasionally cause nausea, pain in the right-hand side of the abdomen below the ribs and **jaundice**.

Brain metastases can present with an epileptic fit due to the tumour irritating the brain. Other symptoms that brain metastases can cause are headaches, weakness of the arms or legs, and sometimes confusion or a change in personality.

Spread to the **adrenal glands** is also quite common, although rarely causes symptoms.

jaundice
Yellow discolouration of the skin and the whites of the eyes due to deposition of bile pigments in the tissues.

adrenal glands
Glands which sit adjacent to the top of the kidneys and produce steroids and adrenaline.

CHAPTER

3

Tests for lung cancer

Tests for lung cancer can be loosely divided into those that are commonly performed in order to make a diagnosis (diagnostic tests) and those that are used to find out how far a lung cancer has spread. These are called staging tests i.e. tests to determine what stage the cancer has reached. However, some tests are used to both diagnose and stage lung cancer.

Most patients who are suspected of having lung cancer are referred by their doctor to a consultant respiratory physician for further investigations. During the first visit a history will be taken and a clinical examination performed. If it has not already been performed, a chest X-ray will usually be taken. The chest X-ray may provide information about which part of the lung is affected. If lung cancer is suspected a CT scan of the lungs and abdomen will usually be performed in order to give further information about the position of the tumour and an initial idea of how far the cancer has spread.

In order to make a diagnosis of lung cancer a **biopsy** of the tumour is usually required. In addition to confirming the diagnosis, a biopsy will give information about the type of lung cancer. This is important in helping to determine the type of treatment that may be offered. Information about the different types of lung cancer is given in Chapter 1.

> **biopsy**
> The removal of a small piece of tissue in order to make a diagnosis.

The most common tests used to take a biopsy are either a bronchoscopy or a CT-guided lung biopsy. The best test to do depends upon the position of the tumour within the lung. If the tumour appears to be accessible from one of the bronchi, it is likely that a bronchoscopy will be offered. If the tumour is lying towards the outside edge of the lung, it is likely that a CT-guided lung biopsy will be recommended. However, not all lung cancers can be biopsied using these techniques and sometimes more specialist techniques are needed.

The exact diagnostic and staging tests that a patient needs is dependent on a number of different factors and your doctor will be able to advise you about which ones are needed in your particular case.

Details about all the different possible diagnostic and staging procedures are given in this chapter. Many hospitals that perform tests such as those outlined here produce comprehensive patient information leaflets which explain why patients are having the test, how it will be done, and what arrangements they should make for their visit to the hospital.

Commonly performed tests for diagnosing and staging lung cancer

CT scan

> **myth**
> Having a CT scan involves being placed inside a long dark tunnel.

> **fact**
> Modern CT scanners are usually housed in large, airy rooms and look a bit like a large doughnut. The vast majority of people do not find them claustrophobic.

A CT scan uses X-rays to build up a three-dimensional picture of the inside of the body. In addition to giving information about the position of the tumour within the lung, a CT scan will often provide information about how far the tumour has spread within the lung and whether it has spread to other parts of the body.

A CT scan involves lying very still on your back on a special table that moves through the scanner during the scan.

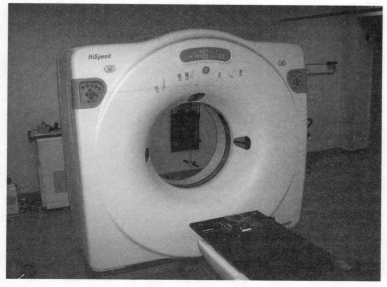

Figure 3.1 A CT scanner. This is used to diagnose and stage lung cancer but can also be used to plan radiotherapy to treat lung cancer.

You may be asked not to eat or drink anything for a few hours before the scan. Most people who have a CT scan to look at the lungs will be given an **intravenous injection** of **contrast** just as the scan is about to start. The contrast will be given through a small tube inserted into a vein in the arm. You may feel a strange, hot, flushing sensation just as the injection is performed. This is quite normal and will pass after a minute or two. If you have asthma or allergies it is important to tell your doctor and the staff doing the CT scan before you have the scan done. Sometimes it is necessary to be given treatment with steroid tablets for a day or two before the test. It is also important to tell the staff who perform the scan if you are diabetic or have kidney disease. If you are on **Metformin** for diabetes you will be asked not to take the drug for two days after the scan. This is because the combination of Metformin and the contrast agent given for the scan can upset kidney function. It may be necessary to check the kidney function with a blood test before you re-start Metformin. The scan itself is painless and takes between ten and 20 minutes. You will be asked to hold your breath for a few seconds while the scan is performed.

intravenous injection
Injection into a vein.

contrast
A special injection of dye given just before a CT scan that outlines the blood vessels and helps the radiologist to identify the blood vessels in the chest.

Metformin
Tablet medication given to some people who have diabetes.

CT-guided lung biopsy

This test is done with the help of a CT scanner. A CT-guided biopsy can be used to either biopsy a mass in the lung or biopsy the pleural lining of the lung if it is thickened and thought to be cancerous. The CT scan is used to identify the best spot for the biopsy. Local anaesthetic is used to freeze the skin on the front or back of the chest before a thin needle is passed through the chest wall into the lung or the pleural lining. The actual biopsy may feel a little uncomfortable and you may feel a pushing sensation when the biopsy is being taken. You may be asked to lie on your front for the biopsy. It is important that you find a comfortable position and lie still during the biopsy process, as sudden movements could cause the needle to damage the lung. Although a lung biopsy is generally a safe procedure there can be some risks associated with it. Occasionally air can leak from the lung through the puncture hole (made by the needle) into the pleural space. This results in a **pneumothorax**.

pneumothorax
Air in the pleural space.

> ### my experience
>
> Following my lung biopsy test the doctors told me that I had developed a small pneumothorax. They explained that this was due to some air which had leaked out of the lung into the space around the lung. I had already noticed that I felt slightly short of breath after the test. The doctors explained that they wanted to keep an eye on the pneumothorax and ensure that it did not get any larger. I was kept in hospital overnight and the following morning had another chest X-ray. This showed that the pneumothorax had not changed so I was allowed to go home. I was told that if I got any more short of breath I was to contact the hospital again and I might need to have the air sucked out with a needle and syringe. I did feel a bit short of breath for a few days but then things improved and when I went back to the clinic the following week the X-ray showed that the pneumothorax had gone.

chest drain
A soft plastic tube that is inserted between the ribs into the pleural space. The drain is usually attached to a one-way underwater seal that allows air or fluid out of the pleural space but does not allow it back in again.

A small pneumothorax after the biopsy is quite common and may need no treatment at all. Occasionally, a large pneumothorax can occur causing breathlessness due to the lung deflating. If this occurs you may need to stay in hospital and have a **chest drain** inserted in order to let the air out of the pleural space and allow the lung to re-inflate. The risk of getting a pneumothorax with a lung biopsy varies from person to person and depends on a number of factors including whether the lungs contain areas of emphysema and where the biopsy is being taken from. The doctors who advise you to have a lung biopsy will be able to give you more information about your particular biopsy and the risk of getting a pneumothorax.

The other complication that can occur is bleeding inside the lung. This is usually fairly minor but does sometimes cause you to cough up small amounts of blood during or after the procedure. The risk of bleeding is a little higher if you are taking aspirin or clopidrogel, and much higher if you are taking warfarin. If you are on any of these blood thinning drugs, your specialist needs to know.

Bronchoscopy

A bronchoscopy test involves passing a slim, flexible telescope through the nose or mouth, down the windpipe (trachea) and into the lungs. It allows the doctor performing the test to inspect the inside of the bronchi and to take samples for analysis in the laboratory. A bronchoscopy is usually performed as a day case procedure. Typically, you will be asked not to eat or drink anything for a few hours before the test. Before the test is performed the back of the throat is sprayed with a local anaesthetic spray and some local anaesthetic jelly is put into the nose which causes the inside of the nose and the back of the throat to go numb. Sedative drugs may be given through a small tube inserted into a vein in the hand or arm. Once you have been made drowsy by the sedation, the doctor will gently insert the bronchoscope through the nostril or mouth and into the trachea. More anaesthetic will be applied to the vocal cords and trachea to minimize coughing. Once inside the lungs the doctor can look around the inside of the airways and take samples if any abnormalities are seen. Various types of biopsies can be taken.

saline solution
Salt water.

Sometimes the inside of the lungs are washed out using a **saline solution**. Biopsies of tumours or the inside of the airways can be taken using a tiny pair of forceps passed down through the bronchoscope. Taking biopsies from inside the lung does not hurt. Sometimes a tumour cannot be seen inside the airways because it is actually lying on the outside of the airway wall. In this case, it is possible to pass a fine needle through the wall of the airway into the tumour or a lymph gland. This is called a transbronchial needle biopsy. The whole procedure takes about 20–30 minutes. About two hours after the test is completed, and once the sedation has worn off, you can return home.

my experience

I was very nervous about having a bronchoscopy. I have always hated anything touching the back of my throat and I did not think that I would be able to let the doctors put a tube down my throat to look into my lungs. In fact it was much better than I thought it would be. Before the test the doctor sprayed some local anaesthetic onto the back of my throat. It did not taste very nice and it made me cough a bit. As the anaesthetic took effect it felt like having a bit of a lump in the back of my throat. The doctors then gave me an injection of a drug into a vein in my arm in order to sedate me during the procedure. The next thing I remember is the doctors and nurses telling me the test was over. I can't really remember anything about it. Apart from having a slightly sore throat for a day or two afterwards, it was fine.

More specialized tests for diagnosis and staging

In addition to the tests discussed previously, it may be necessary for certain patients to undergo further, more specialized tests and procedures in order to make a diagnosis or assess how far a lung cancer has spread. Your doctor will be able to explain which tests you need to undergo and why. Details of these tests are given in the pages that follow.

There are several different types of scans and procedures that may be performed:

✧ PET (positron emission tomography) scan
✧ ultrasound scan
✧ MRI (magnetic resonance imaging) scan
✧ isotope bone scan.

PET (positron emission tomography) scan

PET scans are used to give an idea of how far a cancer has spread. All cells and tissues in the body use **glucose**, absorbed from food that we eat, to work and grow. A PET scan makes use of the fact that different tissues use glucose at different rates. Cancer cells within a tumour often take up glucose more quickly than other tissues around the tumour and therefore show up as an area of increased activity. PET scans can show up not only the primary tumour but also any metastases throughout the body – the exceptions to this are the brain and the heart. The reason for this is that the brain and the heart are constantly working and using glucose so always show up 'hot' on a PET scan. A CT scan or MRI scan is used to examine the brain if spread of cancer is suspected.

> **glucose**
> A type of sugar.

A PET scan involves having an intravenous injection of a special glucose solution containing a small amount of radioactivity. This is allowed to circulate around the body for an hour or so before the scan is performed. The scan itself involves lying still on a scanning table for about an hour. Prior to the injection you will be asked not to eat or drink for several hours and immediately before the injection you will be asked to lie quietly on a bed without talking for an hour or so. This is in order to prevent the muscles in your body, which also use lots of glucose, doing too much work and interfering with the scan results.

Although PET scans can provide a lot of useful information about tumours and their spread, they can sometimes show up hot areas which are not actually due to cancer. This is because other processes such as inflammation and infection can also use glucose and show up positive on the scan. This can result in 'false positive' results. Therefore, having identified any areas on the scan which are positive it is often important to biopsy that area to confirm that it is actually due to cancer rather than a non-cancerous cause.

At present the number of PET scanners in the UK is limited, although recently new guidelines have stated that all lung cancer patients should be able to have a PET scan if necessary. Whereas at present this may mean travelling some distance to the nearest scanner, it is likely that over the next few years many more scanners will be built. Furthermore, some hospitals are currently using mobile scanners which come to the hospital every week or two in a large van. The most recent generation of PET scanners also incorporate a combined CT scan which makes it possible to do a CT–PET scan. The main advantage of this type of scan is that it allows the doctors to identify exactly where the hot spot on the PET scan lies. This is very useful if a biopsy of a hot spot is needed.

Ultrasound scan

Ultrasound uses sound waves to look at the tissues inside the body. Most people are familiar with ultrasound scans which are used to look at the foetus when a woman is pregnant. Although ultrasound uses sound waves, they are of very high frequency and cannot be heard by humans. An ultrasound test is safe, simple and completely painless. After putting some gel on the skin a hand-held transmitter is held firmly on the skin over the area to be scanned. The ultrasound waves bounce off the tissues under the skin and different tissues reflect the sound waves differently. A computer is used to transform the pattern of reflected sound waves into an image.

In lung cancer, an ultrasound scan can be used to look at the liver to try to separate common liver cysts from metastases. It can also be used to identify enlarged lymph glands in the neck and fluid lying in the pleural space around the lung. Ultrasound scanning is also used to help take biopsy samples. Here, the skin is first numbed using a local anaesthetic and then a fine needle is passed into the structure to be biopsied using ultrasound to guide the needle into the correct place.

MRI (magnetic resonance imaging) scan

An MRI scan can be used to study various parts of the body, but in patients with lung cancer the

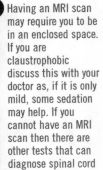

Q I am claustrophobic so can I have an MRI scan?

A Having an MRI scan may require you to be in an enclosed space. If you are claustrophobic discuss this with your doctor as, if it is only mild, some sedation may help. If you cannot have an MRI scan then there are other tests that can diagnose spinal cord compression.

most common areas to be scanned are the brain, the spine and sometimes the bones. MRI scanning uses a strong magnetic field and radiowave signals to produce images of the body. It does not involve any radiation. During an MRI scan you lie on a comfortable padded table which moves inside the scanner. The scanning process is noisy and you will be given earplugs or earphones to wear.

Isotope bone scan

An isotope bone scan (also called a radionuclide scan) involves having an injection of a radioactive fluid (or radionuclide) through a vein in the arm. Then, after a couple of hours, a scan of the whole skeleton is taken using a machine called a gamma camera. The radionuclide travels through the bloodstream and collects in the bones, especially in areas where there is a lot of activity in the bone. These areas of high activity are called hot spots and they show up areas where there is bone breakdown or repair. Hot spots can indicate areas where there are metastases in the bones, but they can also show up areas where there is arthritis or recent fractures. If there are any hot spots found on the bone scan you will usually be asked to have ordinary X-rays taken of the affected area in order to compare them with the results from the bone scan.

Medical procedures

Pleural aspiration

Pleural aspiration involves taking a sample of fluid from a pleural effusion. A suitable site is identified

Q I have recently been having tests for lung cancer. I have had a bronchoscopy test which has shown a lung cancer and the CT scan has shown some fluid around my lung. The doctors now want to take some of this fluid off. Why is this?

A In order to find out how far a lung cancer has spread, it is sometimes necessary to take off fluid that is lying in the pleural space around the lung. This will be examined by a pathologist to see if it contains cancer cells. This will give important information about the stage of the disease and will help to determine the best course of treatment.

either by clinical examination or by using an ultrasound scan to find the fluid. Having numbed the skin with some local anaesthetic, a fine needle is inserted through the skin, between the ribs and into the pleural space. Fluid is sucked out into a syringe for laboratory tests.

Pleural biopsy

A pleural biopsy involves taking a sample of the pleural lining that covers the inside of the rib cage (parietal pleura) (see Figure 1.3). It is usually performed to investigate the cause of a pleural effusion. In order to do this a small incision is made in the skin between the ribs on the affected side under local anaesthetic. A special pleural biopsy needle is then inserted through the hole and several biopsies of the pleural lining are taken. Although the procedure is performed using local anaesthetic, the patient may feel some pressure in the side of the chest as the procedure is being performed. Sometimes an ultrasound scan is used to try to identify the best spot to take the biopsies from. Potential risks from this technique are bleeding at the site of the biopsy and the creation of a pneumothorax. After the procedure a chest X-ray is performed in order to check that a pneumothorax has not occurred.

The main problem with this type of biopsy technique is that it is not always very easy to tell where to take the biopsies from. As a result the biopsies might not show any evidence of cancer even when it is present. For this reason, this type of pleural biopsy is used less frequently nowadays; pleural biopsies are more commonly being performed using a CT scanner to identify the best place to biopsy or by using a technique called thoracoscopy. Further details of these tests are given in this chapter in the section on CT-guided lung biopsy and thoracoscopy respectively.

Endobronchial ultrasound

This is a specialized test that is only available in a few centres in the UK at present although it is likely to become more widely available in the next few years. It allows samples to be taken from the lymph glands in the mediastinum. This is sometimes important for accurate staging of a lung cancer. From the patient's point of view it is very similar to a bronchoscopy test. However, it is performed using a very specialized bronchoscope that has both a camera and a small ultrasound probe at its tip. The camera is used to navigate the bronchoscope around the inside of the airways and the ultrasound probe allows lymph nodes that lie on the outside of the airways to be seen. Biopsies of the lymph nodes can be taken by passing a fine needle out from the end of the scope, through the wall of the airway and into the lymph gland. The images produced by the ultrasound are used to guide the needle into the correct position. The biopsy procedure is painless.

Endoscopic ultrasound

Endoscopic ultrasound is a specialized test that is only available in certain hospitals. It involves passing a thin, flexible telescope (thinner than your little finger) through the mouth, into the gullet (oesophagus), and down into the stomach. At the end of the scope is a light, a camera and a small ultrasound probe.

While the camera is used to look around the inside of the gullet and stomach, the ultrasound probe produces images of the tissues around the outside of the gullet and stomach. On its way to the stomach, the gullet passes through the central area of the chest (mediastinum) and passes close to lymph glands, the heart and the liver. Therefore endoscopic ultrasound can be used to examine the lymph glands in the mediastinum and also to take biopsies from them. This is done by passing a fine needle out from the end of the scope, through the wall of the gullet and into the lymph gland. The images produced by the ultrasound are used to guide the needle into the correct place to take the biopsies. The procedure is done using sedation and the biopsy procedure is painless.

Surgical procedures

Mediastinoscopy

Mediastinoscopy is a surgical operation that is performed to take biopsies of lymph glands from the central part of the chest (see Figure 1.4) in order to find out whether the lung cancer has spread to the lymph nodes or not. It is performed under a general anaesthetic in an operating theatre and involves making a two to three centimetre cut in the hollow at the bottom of the neck, just above the breastbone (sternum) (see Figure 3.2). The surgeon passes a short, metal tube with a light attachment (mediastinoscope) through the incision and down into the chest, just in front of the windpipe (trachea) (see Figure 1.4). This allows access to the lymph glands that lie around the windpipe and biopsies are taken for examination under the microscope. Once the

Q Why has my specialist asked me to have a mediastinoscopy?

A Sometimes it is important to take samples from the lymph glands in the centre of the chest (the mediastinum) in order to find out if a lung cancer has spread there. This may be because the CT scan has shown that some of the glands are enlarged or because one of them has shown up 'hot' on a PET scan. This will give information about whether the lymph glands are affected by cancer and will help to decide what treatment can be offered.

tube is removed, the small cut is sewn up with invisible stitches that dissolve themselves and do not need to be taken out. This is a minor operation and patients are normally able to go home after 24 hours or so.

Although complications are uncommon (in less than one per cent of cases), they can occur. Many of the large blood vessels of the chest lie nearby and if one of them is damaged during the procedure major bleeding can result. Control of such bleeding can usually be stemmed through the same incision but, very rarely, it may be necessary to open the chest through one side or the other, or sometimes through the middle of the breastbone. Occasionally the wound can become infected but this is usually easily treated with a course of antibiotics.

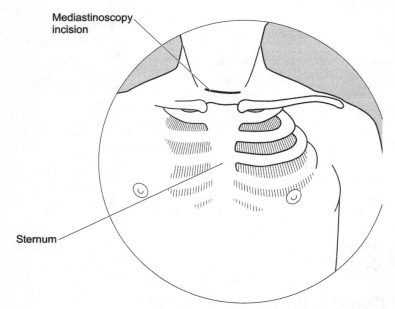

Mediastinoscopy incision

Sternum

Figure 3.2 Position of incision for a mediastinoscopy.

Mediastinotomy

An anterior mediastinotomy operation is another way of biopsying lymph glands in the left side of the chest. Cancers in the left lung can spread to lymph nodes that lie around the arch of the aorta, the main blood vessel that takes blood from the heart to the rest of the body. This area cannot be accessed by a mediastinoscopy and therefore a different approach is required.

Under a general anaesthetic a five to eight centimetre cut is made to the left side of the breastbone about five centimetres above the left nipple (see Figure 3.3). Having separated the tissues of the chest wall, the surgeon can then look into the chest using the mediastinoscope

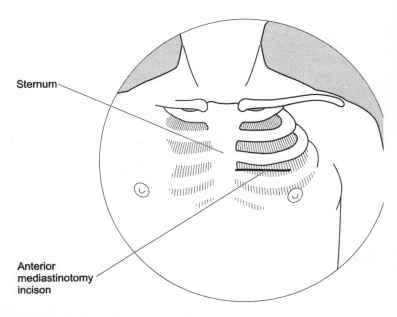

Sternum

Anterior
mediastinotomy
incison

Figure 3.3 Position of incision for an anterior mediastinotomy.

(described earlier in this chapter) and take samples from the lymph glands around the aorta. Once complete the wound is closed with dissolving stitches. Occasionally it may be necessary to leave a drainage tube within the chest to allow any fluid or air that may need draining to escape. If this happens, the tube can usually be removed within 24 to 48 hours. Complications are rare. If they do occur, then the commonest are bleeding and infection.

Thoracoscopy

This is essentially keyhole surgery in the chest. It is used both for taking biopsies to make a diagnosis and also for assessing how far a cancer has spread. Thoracoscopy is sometimes performed as a medical procedure using local anaesthetic and sedation and sometimes as a surgical procedure under a general anaesthetic.

Medical thoracoscopy

The procedure itself involves making a small incision in the chest wall to allow a short telescope-like instrument called a thoracoscope to be inserted into the pleural space around the lung (see Figure 1.3). To do this the lung has to be allowed to collapse – in effect a pneumothorax is created. The pleural space and the pleural lining of the lung can then be inspected. If a pleural effusion is present this can be removed and biopsies of the pleural lining can be taken under direct vision. Being able to see exactly where to take the biopsy from means that this technique often has a much higher success rate for diagnosis than the older, traditional method of taking pleural biopsies. At the end of the procedure a chest drain is inserted through the same hole that was used for the thoracoscope and this is left in place for a day or two until the lung re-expands. Once the lung has re-inflated the drain is removed.

Surgical thoracoscopy

When a thoracoscopy is performed by a surgeon the procedure is often called video-assisted thoracoscopic surgery or VATS (see Figure 3.4). The advantage of performing the procedure under general anaesthetic is that it can allow more extensive biopsy procedures to be performed. In addition to taking biopsies of the pleura, the surgeon can also take biopsies from some lymph glands that lie in the mediastinum or from the actual lung itself. Sometimes lung nodules that are too small or too difficult to biopsy by a CT-guided lung biopsy method can be sampled and checked for cancer during the operation. This is called a **frozen section**.

> **frozen section**
> A biopsy which is frozen immediately after removal and examined during the operation.

If the nodule turns out to be cancerous it can then be removed completely or if it is non-cancerous it can be left alone. However, in order to perform these more complex biopsy procedures using keyhole surgery it is often necessary to make two or three small incisions in the chest wall rather than one. This is to allow the surgeon to put the various surgical instruments inside the chest that he/she needs to perform the operation.

Lung function tests

Lung function tests provide information about how healthy the lungs are and how well they

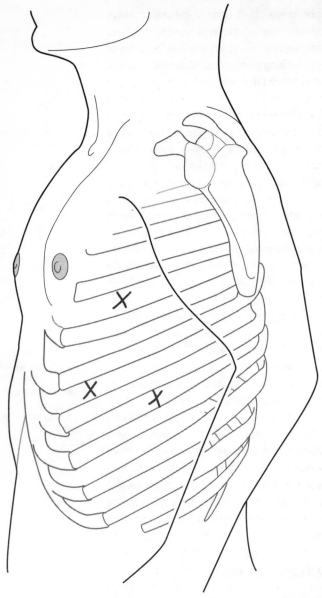

Figure 3.4 Position of incisions for a video-assisted thoracoscopic procedure.

work. The majority of patients with lung cancer are, or have been, cigarette smokers and in addition to having lung cancer they may have chronic bronchitis or emphysema. These conditions affect the health of the lungs and can influence what tests can be done and what treatments are possible. It is particularly important to know how well the lungs are working before contemplating a surgical operation to remove a lung cancer or before giving radiotherapy to the lungs. Lung function tests can vary from quite simple measurements, involving blowing into a plastic tube, to complex assessments which require many measurements and which may take an hour or two to complete. Sometimes walking tests are performed in order to determine how far a patient can walk within a set time.

Getting the results of the tests

Attending a clinic consultation in order to get the results of tests is often a very stressful and worrying experience for many people. In order to make it a bit easier it is a good idea for the patient to ask a friend or relative if they can accompany them. It is well recognized that patients often remember less than half of what they are told in a consultation; if bad news is being broken it is very likely that the patient will remember little of what is said after the initial diagnosis is given. Not only can a friend or relative provide much needed emotional support at a very difficult time but they are far more likely to remember what is said and can take notes and ask questions that the patient may have forgotten. Attending with a written list of questions can be a useful *aide-mémoire*.

When I returned to the lung clinic after my tests I asked one of my best friends if she would come with me. I had suspected that I would be told that I had lung cancer as the doctors had already warned me that that was what they were concerned about. Although I was expecting the diagnosis it still came as a hugh shock to be told 100 per cent that was what it definitely was. I had still been hoping that it would simply be some infection. After the doctor told me I really could not think of anything and I simply remember watching his lips moving but not really hearing what he was saying. All I could think of was that I had lung cancer. When we got home my friend told me all the things that the doctor had said. I still cannot remember him actually saying any of it. The next day I phoned the lung cancer nurse who had been in the room too and she went over the conversation again. Having my friend there was invaluable – I was really surprised how the news affected me at the time.

specialist cancer nurse
An experienced nurse who specializes in the care of patients with cancer.

Some cancer clinics are beginning to tape consultations and give a tape of the discussion to the patient at the end of the meeting so that they can listen to it again at home with family. Other clinics provide written notes of the main issues discussed. At many cancer clinics the consultation will be with a doctor and a **specialist cancer nurse**. The nurse will often be able to go over the main points of the consultation again and answer further questions about diagnosis and treatment. They will also act as a point of contact with the lung cancer team and be able to provide continuity and guidance during subsequent treatment visits.

CHAPTER

4

The surgical treatment of lung cancer

It is well recognized that the surgical removal of a lung cancer offers the best chance of curing the disease. Previous experience has shown that patients with Stage 1 and Stage 2 non-small cell lung cancer (see Chapter 1 for details) are most likely to be cured by surgery. In order to attempt to cure a lung cancer by surgery it is very important to remove the entire tumour together with any affected lymph glands.

If the cancer has spread to the lymph glands at the root of the lung (hilar glands) it is usually possible to remove them along with the main tumour. However, if the tumour has spread to the lymph glands in the centre of the chest (the mediastinum – see Figure 1.4) or if it has started to invade other structures within the chest such as the heart or the major blood vessels it is much less likely that surgery will be able to provide a cure. The reason for this is that it is not usually possible to remove all the affected tissue successfully and invariably the tumour re-occurs following surgery. Therefore, determining the extent of spread of a lung cancer before a surgical operation is essential. This is called 'staging' the cancer and is discussed in Chapter 3.

Occasionally, despite all the staging tests it is not possible to be absolutely sure of the extent of a tumour. In these cases an operation may be offered in the hope that it is possible to remove all of the cancer. However, sometimes this does lead to the situation where the chest is opened but after a thorough inspection it is decided that the cancer is not removable. This unfortunate scenario is called an 'open and close' operation. Although this does still happen in about five per cent of surgical operations it is much less common now than it used to be due to the improvements in the staging tests available. All patients who are having a surgical operation to try to remove a lung cancer should be advised that only when the surgeons examine the inside of the chest will they be able to confirm whether the cancer can be removed or not.

Types of operation used to remove lung cancer

The aim of removing a lung cancer is to completely remove the cancer while sparing as much healthy lung as possible. The most common operation is the removal of a single lobe of a lung (**lobectomy**), provided that the cancer is confined to a single lobe (see Figure 1.2 for a diagram of the lobes of each lung). However, if a tumour crosses into another lobe it may be necessary to remove two lobes (bi-lobectomy). This is quite common if the tumour is lying in the

myth

Having an operation to remove a lung cancer will definitely result in a cure.

fact

Although it has been shown that complete removal of an early stage lung cancer by surgery offers the best chance of cure, it is possible that the cancer could return in the first few years following the operation. This is because sometimes the cancer has spread at an early stage and despite all the currently available pre-operative tests this 'micro-metastatic' disease can not be detected. Sometimes chemotherapy is offered after an operation to try and decrease the chance that the cancer comes back.

lobectomy

The removal of a single lobe of the lung, together with the lymph glands at the root of the lung.

middle lobe of the right lung. Often the right upper lobe or right lower lobe is removed along with the middle lobe. Occasionally, if a tumour is small and lies towards the edge of the lung, the surgeon may remove part but not all of a lobe. This is called a **segmentectomy**. However, sometimes, due to the position or size of a tumour, it may be necessary to remove a whole lung. This is called a **pneumonectomy** operation.

If a patient has limited lung function and will not withstand a standard lobectomy it may be decided to remove a localized area of lung around the tumour. This is called a **wedge resection** (see Figure 4.1). While it is hoped that this approach will affect a cure there is an increased risk that the cancer may reoccur in the part of the lobe that remains.

Sometimes surgery is performed to remove a tumour that is affecting the upper lobe (or middle lobe) and the main bronchus. Instead of removing the whole lung it is sometimes possible to remove the upper or middle lobe and the affected section of the main bronchus and then re-implant the healthy lower lobe onto the remaining healthy main bronchus (see Figure 4.2). This operation is called a **sleeve resection** and allows the lower lobe to be spared thereby retaining as much healthy lung as possible.

In certain circumstances surgeons will attempt to remove more advanced tumours that have spread to lymph glands in the centre of the chest or to other structures such as the diaphragm or the chest wall. This is obviously more extensive surgery and a very careful assessment of the patient has to be made to ensure that they are fit enough to withstand the operation, and any subsequent treatment such as chemotherapy or

segmentectomy
The removal of a segment of a lobe. Each lobe of the lung is composed of several segments.

pneumonectomy
The removal of an entire lung along with the associated lymph glands.

wedge resection
The removal of a small wedge-shaped portion of lung.

sleeve resection
The removal of the upper or middle lobe and affected area of bronchus. The healthy lower lobe is then re-implanted onto remaining healthy bronchus.

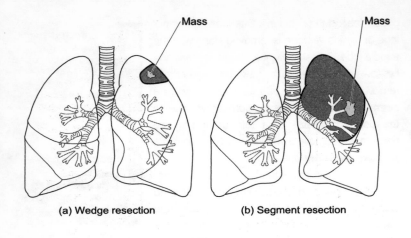

(a) Wedge resection   (b) Segment resection

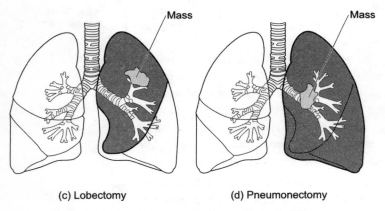

(c) Lobectomy   (d) Pneumonectomy

Figure 4.1 Types of operations used to remove lung cancer.

radiotherapy that may be required. If this type of operation is being considered the surgeon will discuss the benefits and potential risks with the patient in great detail.

During all the operations listed above (except wedge resections) the surgeon will remove the lymph glands that lie at the root of the lung (hilar glands) in addition to as many of the mediastinal lymph nodes that can be found. The actual lymph

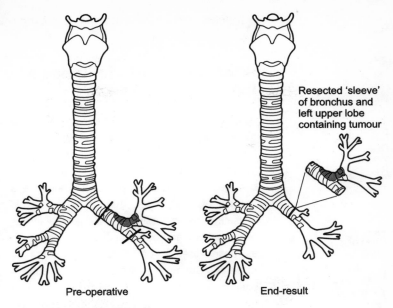

Resected 'sleeve'
of bronchus and
left upper lobe
containing tumour

Pre-operative

End-result

▌ Figure 4.2 A sleeve resection.

glands removed will vary on whether the upper,
middle or lower lobe is being removed. The
lymph glands will be examined by the pathologist
to help determine how far the cancer has spread
and whether it has all been removed.

Sometimes surgeons will send samples of
tissue to the pathologist during the operation in
order to find out whether the tissue contains
cancer or not. It is not always easy for the surgeon
to determine exactly how far the cancer has
spread just by looking at it. In order to check
whether tissue contains cancer or not a small
piece is taken out and immediately frozen by the
pathologist. Very thin slices are then taken and
examined under the microscope. This is called
taking a frozen section (see Chapter 3). The
pathologist can then help the surgeon decide
how much tissue to remove in order to

completely remove the tumour but not cut out too much healthy lung.

What are the risks of having a lung cancer operation?

All major operations carry a risk of dying. Normally this is quite low and in general the risk of dying as a result of a lobectomy is between one and two per cent. For a pneumonectomy the risk is higher, between one and eight per cent. There are a number of other factors that can alter the risk. These include: increasing age; the general fitness of the patient; and other medical problems such as heart disease, bronchitis, emphysema or diabetes. During the assessment for surgery patients are carefully assessed for risk. Prior to surgery the surgeon will also discuss the potential risks involved with the patient. Quite often other tests such as an **echocardiogram**, **coronary angiography** or detailed lung function tests may be required in order to assess how well the heart and lungs are working. Sometimes it is necessary to perform coronary artery interventions prior to lung surgery in order to decrease the risk of having a heart attack at the time of the operation.

echocardiogram
An ultrasound test to look at the heart and the tissues surrounding it.

coronary angiography
An X-ray picture of the blood vessels that supply the heart muscle. A fine, hollow tube called a catheter is inserted into an artery in the forearm or groin and advanced through the blood vessels until it reaches the heart. A dye is then injected into the blood vessels and X-rays taken from several angles which provides a 'road map' of the vessels supplying the heart (coronary arteries). Any narrowings of the coronary arteries can be assessed.

my experience

Following my diagnosis of lung cancer the doctors suggested that I might be able to have an operation to remove it. However, because of the chest pains that I had also been getting, I initially had an angiogram performed. This showed that the main blood vessels supplying my heart were narrowed. My heart specialist recommended that I have a coronary artery bypass operation. After this my angina stopped and I was able to go ahead with my lung operation.

Where is the incision made and how large will it be?

The most common site for entry to the chest is through the side of the chest around and below the shoulder blade (scapula) (see Figure 4.3). This is called a postero-lateral thoracotomy. **'Thoracotomy'** simply means making an opening in the chest. Postero-lateral describes the site of the incision – behind (posterior) and to the side (lateral). A standard thoracotomy incision is usually about 15–25 centimetres long. A very common misconception is that the surgeon will break the ribs to enter the chest. This is not the case.

Once the skin has been incised, the muscles beneath are separated, taking care to cut them as little as possible. There are two main layers of muscles that need to be separated before reaching the chest wall itself. Each rib is joined to the one above and the one below by three layers of muscles called the intercostal muscles. These muscles are carefully, but deliberately, separated from the rib either at the upper part of the space to be entered or at the lower part.

The exact rib space chosen by the surgeon for the thoracotomy depends upon the part of the lung that needs to be reached. The upper and middle lobe on the right and the upper lobe on the left are best accessed through an opening between the fifth and sixth ribs. Sometimes in a tall patient the lower lobes can best be removed through the sixth and seventh rib space. To reduce the pressure upon the ribs as they are gently eased apart, in order to get into the chest cavity, it may be necessary to remove a small section of a rib. This is only one to two

thoracotomy
A surgical procedure to open up the chest.

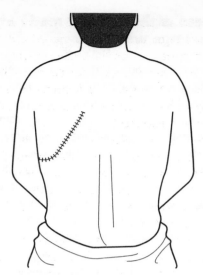

◗ Figure 4.3 Position of a thoracotomy incision.

centimetres long and is not in any way detrimental to the healing or structure of the chest after the operation. This prevents breakage of ribs in the vast majority of patients.

Video-assisted thoracoscopic surgery (VATS)

This is minimally invasive (keyhole) surgery in the chest. It involves making two to three small (three to five centimetre) incisions in the chest wall between the ribs through which a telescopic camera and various instruments can be placed in order to perform the operation (see Figure 3.4). VATS operations are less intrusive and result in much smaller scars. However, visibility and access for the surgeon is reduced and occasionally, if there is a problem and better access or visibility is required, a VATS operation has to be converted to a traditional thoracotomy. VATS surgery is only available in certain centres in the UK and only certain operations can be performed using this approach. Furthermore, not all patients are suited to having VATS surgery. The surgeon will be able to explain the operation in more detail if this is the chosen treatement.

When the operation is complete and the affected part of the lung has been removed, the chest is closed. One or two tube drains are placed within the chest cavity in order to drain any air or fluid that accumulates in the pleural space around the lung. The tube drains are attached to a drainage bottle that is connected to a vacuum suction to help the remaining lung re-expand again properly after the operation. If a pneumonectomy has been performed some surgeons do not leave any drains in at all; others leave one drain in for a day or so. The muscle layers of the chest are carefully sewn together with strong stitches of a type that will eventually be absorbed. The stitches used to close the skin are most often absorbable sutures placed underneath the skin. They also dissolve although occasionally, as the healing process proceeds, they may be expelled from the skin. This can be a source of concern for patients if they are not expecting this to happen.

Recovery from an operation

Most patients will be nursed on the surgical ward after an operation. However, some patients may spend a period of time in the intensive (critical) care unit until they are well enough to return to the ward. This will likely depend on the type of operation and whether the patient has other medical conditions such as heart disease that requires intensive monitoring post-operatively.

Pain control after an operation

Good pain control after an operation is very important as it helps the patient to breathe deeply and move more easily, which aids recovery. There are several different methods that can be used and prior to the operation the anaesthetist will often discuss the best method of providing pain relief. A commonly used technique is an epidural infusion. This involves the placement of a fine **cannula** in the patient's back into the space around the spinal cord. Through this tube a strong painkiller and a local anaesthetic drug can be given which deadens the nerves that supply the area around the surgical incision. This will usually render the patient pain free during the most painful time in the early days after the operation.

> **cannula**
> A thin, hollow tube used to introduce fluid (or medication) to, or remove it from, the body.

Another method is to inject local anaesthetic around the intercostal nerves themselves. This can be done at the time of the operation, before closing the chest, and then repeated afterwards on the ward. A cannula can be left in the space beneath the pleura (the lining of the chest wall) at the time of surgery and local anaesthetic can be infused into this area for several days after the operation. This gives excellent local pain control.

Finally many surgeons commonly inject local anaesthetic directly into the wound edges and around the drains at the end of the procedure. Again, this can be repeated in the ensuing days after the operation.

my experience

I was very worried before I went for my operation that I would be in a lot of pain afterwards. Before the operation the anaesthetist and the nurses talked to me about the different ways that they could control the pain. I decided to have an epidural anaesthetic. This worked really well for the first couple of days after the operation. After it was removed I was given tablets to control the pain, initially strong opiate-based ones and later paracetamol. These worked well and during the first few weeks I was able to slowly decrease them. The main side-effect of the painkillers was constipation and I was given a laxative by the nurses. My wound is not painful at all now although I do have a slightly numb patch of skin at the front of my chest. The surgeon told me that this is because some of the nerves supplying this area of skin were damaged when the cut was made to open my chest. Hopefully this will improve with time.

More general pain control can be obtained with drugs given into a vein (**intravenous**). One way of doing this is called patient-controlled analgesia or PCA. This involves the patient pressing a button on a small pump which then delivers a controlled amount of painkiller. Regular assessment of the patient's pain and programming of the PCA pump reduces the risk of the patient overdosing on the painkiller. Other drugs that are given by mouth can be given in combination with this if necessary.

In the first few days after the operation the patient's pain control will be monitored carefully by the doctors and nurses on the ward. As the wound begins to heal and the patient becomes more active again the amount of painkillers required will decrease. However, it is usual for the patient to be sent home with pain-killing tablets which should be reduced gradually as time passes. Pain relief is a very personal thing and the most appropriate method will vary from patient to patient. It is usual that the team of

Q How long will I spend in hospital for my operation?

A The length of time that you will have to spend in hospital depends upon a number of factors including the type of operation that you are having, your general level of fitness before the operation and whether there are any complications. Generally speaking, patients having a lobectomy may expect to be in hospital for 5–7 days and those having a pneumonectomy 7–10 days. Patients having a diagnostic or staging procedure such as a mediastinoscopy can expect to be out of hospital within a day or two of the operation. Your surgeon will be able to give you a better idea of the time you can expect to be in hospital, based on your particular operation and circumstances.

intravenous
A drug given directly into a vein via a small sterile tube or cannula.

doctor, nurse and patient will arrive at a combination of methods that work best for the individual patient.

Removal of drains

The drains that are left in the chest after the operation are there to drain fluid and air from around the lung. During the removal of the lung, although the individual lobes of the lung have their own blood supplies and airways, the actual lung tissue (the parenchyma), is often continuous between lobes. Therefore, during the operation they have to be separated. This often results in a leak of air from the cut surface which may take several days to heal. The drains allow this air to escape. Once the lung has started to heal, fluid drainage is less than 100 millilitres every 24 hours and when air stops coming out through the drains it is usually possible to remove them. Removing the drains may be uncomfortable for a short time but painkillers are given beforehand.

Wound healing

The surgical wound is extremely strong from the outset. It has more than enough strength to withstand the normal movements of a patient after the operation. The normal healing process is very rapid. However, for the first six weeks after the operation patients should try to avoid excessive movement around the chest (for example, patients are advised not to play golf or to drive). After this time healing is 90 per cent complete and all normal activities can resume.

Mobilization

Getting going again as soon as possible after the operation is very important. Prior to the operation the nurses and physiotherapists will usually explain and demonstrate breathing and coughing exercises that can be safely performed in the first few days after the operation. These are very important in order to help keep the lungs fully inflated and to prevent the build up of secretions within the lungs. A build up of secretions in the airways can allow infections to develop which at best will slow recovery and at worst could be life threatening. Good pain control will also make deep breathing more comfortable.

Starting on the first day after the operation the nurses and physiotherapists will encourage mobilization. At first it will be gentle arm and leg exercises to prevent stiffness and help the circulation. From the second or third day after the operation patients are helped to get up and about. Until full mobility is regained it is common practice for injections of a blood-thinning drug to be given and anti-thrombosis stockings to be worn. This helps to prevent a **deep vein thrombosis (DVT)** from developing.

Resuming activity

Lung cancer operations are major operations and recovery usually takes some weeks or months. Recovery times are often dependent upon how fit and well the patient was before the operation. Not surprisingly younger patients usually recover more quickly than older patients. For the first two to three weeks light activities only (light housework, weeding the garden) are recommended. More

> **deep vein thrombosis (DVT)**
> A blood clot that can develop in one of the large veins inside the leg or pelvis.

strenuous activities such as carrying shopping, mowing the lawn, digging the garden are not advisable for six to eight weeks after discharge. Sexual intercourse can be resumed once the patient feels confident to do so. Adopting a more passive role may help the return to a normal routine.

About six weeks after discharge patients are normally reviewed in the out-patients clinic by the surgical team. At this visit issues such as resumption of driving and return to work will be discussed. Flying is not recommended until this review has taken place.

Complications following lung surgery

Although the majority of lung operations go smoothly complications can, and do, happen occasionally.

Bleeding

Occasionally bleeding occurs in the chest after the operation and the chest has to be re-opened in order to stop the bleeding. This is an uncommon complication.

Infection

Several types of infection can occur following surgery. The most common and least serious are wound infections which can usually be treated with antibiotic tablets. A chest infection is a more serious complication, the risk of which is exacerbated by poor pain control that limits deep breathing and coughing in the post-operative period. An inability to cough and breathe deeply can lead to sputum retention in the airways. Good pain control and physiotherapy will be used to prevent this from happening. Occasionally an infection can develop in the pleural space around the lung. This is called an **empyema**. Treatment entails drainage of the pus using carefully placed drains in conjunction with antibiotics. Occasionally it is necessary to leave a drain in place for several weeks or months after the operation. If this is necessary it is usually possible to have a short drain connected to a bag so that the patient can get dressed, move around and even return home with the drain in place.

empyema
Pus in the pleural space around the lung.

Deep vein thrombosis and pulmonary embolus

Any period of immobility can result in the development of a deep vein thrombosis in a leg vein or in one of the veins in the pelvis. If the thrombus becomes detached it can travel through the veins and lodge in the heart or the lungs. If this happens it is called a pulmonary embolus. This is a serious complication which can be life threatening. Around the time of the operation heparin injections will normally be administered in order to try to minimize the risk of this occurring. In addition, early mobilization following the operation will help to prevent this problem.

Bronchopleural fistula

During the removal of a lobe of lung or an entire lung the airway to the diseased part of the lung has to be closed off before the lung can be removed. If after the operation the sewn up

fistula
Abnormal connection
between two parts of
the body.

stump breaks down an air leak between the remaining airway and the pleural space can develop. This is called a bronchopleural **fistula**. This sometimes happens if there is any infection in the stump or in the pleural space. If this does happen then treatment is dependent upon the size of the fistula. Sometimes glue can be used to seal a small fistula but occasionally a further operation is required to repair the leak.

Post-thoracotomy neuralgia

At the time of surgery there is inevitably some damage to the intercostal nerves that supply the muscles, tissues and skin between the ribs. Occasionally after the operation these nerves can cause an aching pain in the chest wall. This may be associated with a pins and needles sensation around the front end of the wound and beyond the front end of the incision. There may be a numb area around the middle of the incision as the nerve to that central area is not working at all and the unpleasant sensations are arising from the nerves above and below the space that has been entered. It is more common if pain control has not been good in the early days after the operation or if the patient has suffered a significant wound infection resulting in chronic inflammation around the nerves. Management of this condition can be difficult and may require help from a pain specialist. In a few unfortunate patients this problem can last for several years.

Q What is a multidisciplinary meeting?

A This is a (usually weekly) meeting in which cancer specialists get together to discuss the investigation and management of each patient with lung cancer. The meeting often consists of chest physicians, oncologists, thoracic surgeons, radiologists, pathologists, palliative care specialists and specialist lung cancer nurses. Further information about the multidisciplinary lung cancer team is given in Chapter 9.

Additional treatments

After the operation a pathologist will examine the lung, lymph nodes and other structures that have been removed. This examination will give the final tumour staging. These findings will usually be discussed at the multi-disciplinary meeting. If there has been any tumour left behind post-operative radiotherapy may be recommended. In some cases post-operative (**adjuvant**) chemotherapy may be recommended (see Chapter 6 for further information).

adjuvant
Treatment which is given in addition to the main treatment.

CHAPTER

5

Radiotherapy

What is radiotherapy?

Radiotherapy or radiation therapy is a widely used treatment for cancers including lung cancer. Radiotherapy involves the use of ionizing radiation, usually high energy X-rays, to kill cancer cells which make up tumours. Radiotherapy is usually given externally which means that X-ray beams (photons) are aimed at the tumour from a machine called a linear accelerator (linac) (see Figure 5.1). There are a number of factors which go into working out how radiotherapy is best given.

Radiotherapy planning

To give treatment effectively the tumour needs to be targeted whilst protecting the surrounding normal tissues as much as possible. In order to do this, treatment needs to be planned and

Q How does radiation kill tumour cells?

A Radiation enters the cell and damages the DNA in the nucleus of the cell. Normal cells are a little better at repairing the damage to DNA than cancer cells. When a damaged cell comes to divide into two cells the damage to the DNA means that it cannot do so and so the cell dies.

simulated. Virtually all patients having radiotherapy will have to attend for radiotherapy planning before their treatment begins. Patients have to attend a **simulator** session where they will have X-rays taken of the tumour on a machine that looks like a linear accelerator or have a CT scan of the area to be treated (see Figure 3.1). In order to reproduce the positioning of the treatment, patients may have a small permanent mark made under the skin (tattoo), which is about the size of a pin-head. This allows the **radiation oncologist** to define the position of the tumour and area for treatment and also to ensure that other areas, such as the healthy lung, the heart and spinal column, are protected from radiation. The radiation oncologist uses the information

simulator

A machine which mimics the linear accelerator but takes diagnostic X-rays so that the details can be checked before starting treatment on the linear accelerator.

radiation oncologist

A doctor who specializes in radiation therapy to cancers. Sometimes known in the UK as a clinical oncologist.

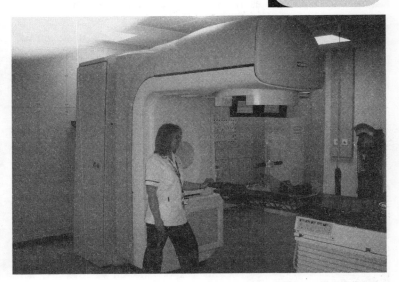

Figure 5.1 A linear accelerator. This machine delivers high energy X-rays. Patients lie on a couch under the machine. A special head and arm rest is used to help keep patients still and in the correct position during treatment.

from the simulator as well as information from other scans and tests. Once the position has been defined a **medical physicist** works out an arrangement of radiation beams best suited to treating the tumour. There may then be an additional appointment a few days later prior to starting treatment to verify that the radiation beams are correctly aimed at the tumour.

medical physicist
A scientist specially trained in the use of radiation to treat tumours.

Treatment

Information from the planning process is transferred directly to the linear accelerator. **Radiographers** deliver treatment on the linear accelerator. Patients will be carefully placed on the linear accelerator in exactly the same position as they were for the planning session.

radiographer
An individual trained to plan and administer radiation therapy.

The length of treatment, number of sessions or **fractions** and complexity of the treatment will be decided depending on the size and stage of the tumour as well as other factors including how able the patient is to tolerate the side-effects of treatment.

fraction
The term given to a single radiotherapy treatment.

After correct positioning the radiographers leave the room and treatment is monitored by closed circuit television. The linear accelerator will move around to treat from different directions. Treatment normally takes around 10 to 15 minutes and is usually once per day during the week with a break at weekends.

radical treatment
A treatment aimed at curing the cancer.

The number of fractions can vary from as few as one or two to over 30. Generally the number of fractions will depend on whether the aim of treatment is to eradicate the tumour (**radical treatment**) or to relieve symptoms (**palliative treatment**). A small number of fractions in a course of treatment usually means

palliative treatment
A treatment which is not designed to cure but to help alleviate or prevent symptoms.

that treatment is designed to help control specific symptoms; longer courses of treatment, such as 20 fractions or over, are given when the intention of treatment is to eradicate the tumour.

Side-effects

Side-effects can be divided into two categories – early side-effects that occur during or in the first few weeks after completion of radiotherapy, and late effects that manifest months and sometimes years after the end of treatment. Most radiotherapy side-effects relate to the part of the body where radiotherapy is being given. One exception to this is general tiredness; this is very common and can last for up to six weeks after completing treatment.

When radiation therapy is given to the lung the other organs that can be affected include the healthy parts of the lung, the heart, the oesophagus (or gullet), the spinal cord (or column) and overlying skin.

Acute side-effects to the skin causing redness and breakdown of the skin are rare nowadays due to the very high energy of X-rays used which pass straight through the skin. The main acute side-effects tend to involve the oesophagus which can become inflamed. Symptoms related to this can include pain or difficulty in swallowing, which is usually worse with lumpy or solid food. If this is the case a semi-solid or liquid diet may be required. In most cases soluble painkillers or indigestion mixtures can be helpful. In very rare cases it is necessary to have liquids given intravenously if the patient is totally unable to swallow.

A mild cough and breathlessness can occur during treatment but if tiredness and breathlessness are more severe the radiation

myth
After radiotherapy I will be radioactive and have to stay away from children and pregnant women.

fact
This form of radiotherapy uses high energy X-rays which are not radioactive. After treatment there are no restrictions on contact with children or others.

acute side-effects
Side-effects which occur during or immediately after treatment.

oncologist should check for anaemia as this can make radiotherapy less effective and can be corrected by a blood transfusion.

Later side-effects can include inflammation of the lung (pneumonitis) which can lead to infection or scarring that can cause breathlessness. It is now possible for radiation oncologists to predict how common this might be by working out how much radiation the healthy parts of the lung will get. Pneumonitis can be helped by a short course of antibiotics or steroids. Very rare late side-effects can include damage to the spinal cord causing paralysis but with modern radiotherapy planning systems this should be an extremely small risk.

When is radiotherapy given?

Radiotherapy is widely used in the treatment of all types of lung cancer. The two main types of lung cancer are non-small cell lung cancer (NSCLC) which accounts for around 80 per cent of lung cancers and small cell lung cancer (SCLC) which makes up the remainder of lung cancers. Other factors such as the stage of the tumour (how far it has spread) and the general fitness and health of the patient will determine whether radiotherapy is appropriate and which type should be given.

Treatment for non-small cell lung cancer (NSCLC)

Radical radiotherapy

Radical radiotherapy is usually recommended when a tumour is technically removable by surgery but there may be a reason, usually medical, why it would not be safe to do so. Many patients with lung cancer have other medical conditions that may make it more difficult for them to undergo a surgical operation. Common conditions where this may be the case include severe bronchitis or emphysema, severe coronary artery disease or other heart disease. In most cases the medical team will make an assessment of a patient's fitness for surgery or radical radiotherapy and discuss the pros and cons of the particular treatment with them.

The level of risk for a treatment will vary from person to person. A person may be fit for surgery but may decide that they do not want an operation and opt for radical radiotherapy. Patients with Stage 1 or 2 disease can be offered radical radiotherapy. The radiotherapy is planned and given over four to six weeks. Typical doses range from 55 **Gray** (Gy) in 20 fractions to 64 Gy in 32 fractions. The exact number of treatments given depends on the volume of tissue that needs to be treated and, to a certain extent, on local practice.

gray
A Gray (Gy) is a unit of radiation dose.

Continuous hyperfractionated accelerated radiotherapy (CHART)

CHART is a radiotherapy regime developed in the UK that is available in certain radiotherapy departments. CHART involves having radiotherapy three times a day, typically 8:00 a.m, 2:00 p.m and 8:00 p.m, with six hours in between treatment fractions. Treatment is given continuously for 12 days with no breaks for weekends. For example, treatment may start on a Monday morning and continue through to the Friday evening of the following week. Therefore, in total 36 fractions are given. The theory behind this type of treatment is that by reducing the time between treatments and the overall treatment time, the tumour cells have less time to grow and divide (repopulation) during the treatment period.

In order that the late effects on the normal tissues (spinal cord, lungs and oesophagus) are not increased, the amount of radiation in each fraction is decreased and the total number of treatments is increased. The acute side-effects of treatment may be more severe with CHART but they do not start until after the treatment is completed and they are generally manageable. As treatment is given continuously over 12 days most patients need to be admitted to hospital or stay in a hostel close to the radiotherapy department.

CHART has been compared to standard daily radiotherapy in a clinical trial and was found to be superior. However, this trial was done several years ago and it is not clear whether CHART is better than the latest radiotherapy regimens. In addition, we do not know whether CHART is better than radiotherapy combined with chemotherapy. Further research is needed in this area.

Chemo-radiotherapy

Radical radiotherapy can be combined in various ways with chemotherapy, and by combining these treatments they can be more effective. The main methods of combining the treatments are:

✧ sequential chemoradiotherapy– where chemotherapy is given first and then followed by radiotherapy

✧ concurrent chemoradiotherapy– when the treatments are given at the same time

The addition of chemotherapy may improve the results of treatment by treating areas of cancer which have spread but are too small to be seen by conventional tests or scans (**micro-metastatic disease**). Each type of chemo-radiotherapy has potential advantages and disadvantages.

Sequential treatment

Sequential treatment allows chemotherapy to take effect and shrink down a tumour before radiotherapy is given. The area of lung which then requires radiotherapy can be smaller and may allow a higher dose of radiation to be given. A disadvantage is that it delays the start of radiotherapy.

> **micro-metastatic disease**
> Disease which has spread in an amount so small it cannot be seen by conventional scans or blood tests.

my experience

After I had all my tests my doctor referred me to an oncologist. As my cancer had not spread outside the chest, but was too advanced for an operation, I was offered a combination of chemotherapy and radiotherapy. The chemotherapy was quite tough but it did help some of my symptoms, particularly my cough. The radiotherapy part was much easier although after all the treatment was completed I had to liquidize my food for a few weeks as I had difficulty swallowing. Also, I was exhausted for about five to six weeks afterwards. I would say it took about two to three months for me to fully recover from the treatment.

Concurrent treatment

Concurrent treatment allows both treatments to be given together, and this has the advantage that chemotherapy can make cancer cells more sensitive to radiation. The disadvantage is that non-cancer cells are also sensitized to radiation and side-effects can be more marked. Platinum-containing drugs (cisplatin and carboplatin) are commonly used and may be combined with other drugs such as etoposide, vinorelbine and docetaxel (see Chapter 6). The dose of these drugs may be lower when they are given with radiotherapy as compared to when they are given on their own. When chemotherapy is given concurrently, chemotherapy drugs can be given at different intervals, for example, every day, every week or every three weeks.

Post-operative radiotherapy

Radiotherapy can be given after surgery for lung cancer, but there are only a few circumstances where it is recommended. Recent research has shown that when a tumour has been completely removed post-operative radiotherapy is not beneficial. Radiotherapy may be indicated when there is evidence that the tumour has not been completely removed or lymph nodes within the mediastinum (N2 disease) show deposits of tumour. In order to define the area to be treated the radiation oncologist will usually need to discuss potential sites of remaining disease with the surgeon, pathologist and radiologist. A course of post-operative radiotherapy typically lasts four to six weeks.

Palliative radiotherapy

Palliative radiotherapy is given with the intention of relieving specific symptoms when lung cancer is at an advanced stage and a cure is not possible. This sort of treatment can be given either to the primary cancer within the chest or to areas where the disease has spread to and is causing symptoms. The planning process is simpler and the number of fractions is less.

Palliative radiotherapy to the primary tumour in the lung or affected lymph nodes in the chest can be effective in alleviating symptoms such as a cough, coughing up blood (haemoptysis), chest pain and sometimes breathlessness. Treatment can be given in as little as one or two treatments or fractions, as research has shown that this is as effective as five or ten fractions, especially when the disease has spread to other areas of the body or patients are frail. If the lung cancer is inoperable but has not spread and the patient is fitter, then treatments may be spread over two to three weeks (10 to 13 fractions). This may give slightly better results. Side-effects of palliative treatment are generally less marked but some patients report flu-like symptoms a few days after treatment, especially if only one or two fractions are given.

Metastatic disease

Lung cancer can spread to other areas of the body. Common sites of spread are to bones, lymph nodes outside the chest and the brain. Radiotherapy can be effective in helping to control pain caused by the spread of disease to the bones and in reducing swelling in lymph nodes outside the chest, usually in the neck. Treatment for this sort of spread is usually given in one to five daily fractions.

Brain metastasis

When lung cancer spreads to the brain it can cause a number of symptoms such as headache, confusion, weakness, loss of balance and visual disturbances. Brain metastases are usually diagnosed by a CT or MRI scan. Tumours in the brain cause the brain to swell and because the brain is contained within the bony box of the skull, the swelling increases the pressure in the brain. Steroids (usually dexamethasone) can be effective in quickly reducing the pressure within the brain. If there is only one isolated metastasis and the disease is controlled in other parts of the body, **neurosurgery** to remove the tumour may be considered. This is usually followed by a course of radiotherapy. However, it is more common for there to be more than one metastasis present and therefore the whole of the brain tissue is treated with radiotherapy. Radiotherapy may be useful but care needs to be taken in assessing the advantages of radiotherapy over the disadvantages which include hair loss, nausea, headaches and tiredness. The best results are seen in patients who are aged less than 60 years of age, have fewer tumours and have the disease stabilized in other areas of the body. To help radiotherapy to the brain to be delivered with accuracy, the patient may have to have a mould or mask made to keep the head in one position during treatment. Commonly two, five or ten fractions are given according to local practice.

Stereotactic radiotherapy, sometimes called radiosurgery or gamma knife treatment is a special type of radiotherapy which can be given as an alternative to surgery or when a tumour returns after radiotherapy has been given. It involves a very high dose of radiation being given which is intensely focused on a very small part of the brain. It is usually reserved for small isolated metastasis.

neurosurgery
Surgery on the brain or the spinal cord.

stereotactic radiotherapy
A type of highly focused radiotherapy where the radiation beams are directed at a small tumour deposit.

Six months after my father completed chemotherapy for his lung cancer he started to get headaches and was unsteady on his feet. A scan showed that the cancer had spread to the brain in at least three areas. He was started on steroids which helped a bit but he was not really himself. Other tests showed that the cancer was returning in the chest as well. The oncologist explained that his life expectancy was going to be a few months and that radiotherapy to the brain was likely to cause a lot of side-effects. Dad decided that he wanted to spend time at home and decided not to have radiotherapy. I was pleased that he did not have unnecessary treatment and he died six weeks later with us all at home.

Brachytherapy

Brachytherapy (or interstitial radiotherapy) is a different type of radiotherapy which involves placing a radioactive source adjacent to the tumour for a period of time. The advantage of this type of treatment is that the tumour can receive a very high dose of radiation with less damage to the surrounding tissues. The main disadvantage is that to place the radioactive source near to the tumour requires a bronchoscopy (see Chapter 3).

Brachytherapy for lung cancer may be used in three ways:

✧ to supplement radical radiotherapy (a boost) to the tumour
✧ as a palliative treatment
✧ when external beam palliative treatment has been given and symptoms have returned, for example, coughing up blood (haemoptysis), and further external beam radiotherapy may risk damaging normal tissues.

Brachytherapy is usually given by an 'after-loading' machine (described later). Firstly, the patient has a bronchoscopy to localize the tumour and a thin hollow tube is passed down through the bronchoscope so that it sits next to the tumour. The tube extends up the airway and out of the nostril. The bronchoscope is then removed leaving the tube in place. The tube is then connected to the after-loading machine which sends a small radioactive pellet on a fine wire down the tube to the tumour. After a few minutes the pellet is removed again by the machine. The thin tube is then also removed from the patient. The patient is only radioactive while the radioactive pellet is inside them. The treatment is performed in a special treatment room. After the treatment is finished the patient can return home. Because the patient is no longer radioactive, no special precautions need to be taken.

Treatment for small cell lung cancer (SCLC)

Chemo-radiotherapy

Around one-third of patients with small cell lung cancer will have a disease which is confined to one side of the chest or thorax. This is known as limited stage disease and, if a patient is fit enough, chemo-radiotherapy is recommended. In small cell lung cancer there is a high risk that the disease can spread to other parts of the body, even if there is no evidence of this from blood tests or scans (micro-metastatic disease) and chemotherapy is the treatment of choice as it can attack cancer in all parts of the body. In limited stage disease, radiotherapy to the tumour and associated lymph glands in the middle of the chest (mediastinum) when added to chemotherapy can sometimes give long-term remission and occasionally cure small cell lung cancer.

In limited stage small cell lung cancer radiotherapy is given during the course of chemotherapy. The exact timing of the radiotherapy can vary but, if possible, it is given early in the course of chemotherapy, for example, with the second or third cycle of chemotherapy. If the tumour is too large or the patient is too frail to cope with treatment at the same time radiotherapy may be given at the end of the chemotherapy. Radiotherapy usually lasts for between three and five weeks (15–25 fractions) during chemotherapy. Recent research has shown that there may be an advantage to receiving radiotherapy twice daily during chemotherapy but further research is ongoing to clarify this.

Prophylactic cranial irradiation (PCI)

Small cell lung cancer tends to spread to other areas of the body readily – particularly, the brain. Chemotherapy will attack the cancer in most parts of the body but the brain is a relatively 'protected' site which means that chemotherapy does not penetrate into the brain as well as other parts of the body. This is sometimes referred to as the blood-brain barrier. Small cell lung cancer can spread to the brain in up to 50 per cent of cases. In limited stage small cell lung cancer it has been shown that giving radiotherapy to the brain in a preventative way can reduce the chance of cancer spreading to the brain to around 20 per cent. PCI is usually recommended when there has been a good response to chemo-radiotherapy and is given towards the end of a course of treatment. However, there are side-effects associated with PCI so it is not routinely given when the disease is more widespread.

If cancer has spread to the brain, the whole brain has to be given radiotherapy as the disease could affect any part. A patient may need to have a special mould or face mask made which they will wear during the radiotherapy sessions to help keep their head in one fixed position for the treatment. Treatment is usually planned and lasts for around two weeks. Acute side-effects can include headache, nausea and extended hair loss after chemotherapy. Tiredness, especially after chemotherapy, can be severe and may even be delayed for a few weeks after treatment has been completed. In the past there have been concerns that PCI could have longer term effects on concentration and memory but research seems to suggest that this can be an effect of the cancer itself in some people rather than the treatment.

Palliative radiotherapy

In around two-thirds of cases there is definite evidence that small cell lung cancer has spread to other parts of the body and this is called extensive stage disease. The usual treatment for this is chemotherapy but radiotherapy can be used as an alternative treatment, either when chemotherapy has not worked or when a patient is felt to be too frail to withstand chemotherapy.

Radiotherapy can also be used when small cell lung cancer is pressing on the main blood vessel taking blood from the upper part of the body to the heart. This causes superior vena cava obstruction (SVCO). It is also used to when small cell lung cancer is causing symptoms due to spread to other parts of the body, for example, bones, and lymph glands in the neck and the brain. Radiotherapy is usually a short course of up to five fractions.

CHAPTER

6

Chemotherapy

What is chemotherapy?

Chemotherapy is a form of systemic or whole body treatment for cancers, including lung cancer. There are many different types of chemotherapy or **cytotoxic drugs**, but they all act in a similar way by killing cells. They are used in cancer treatment to kill cancer cells because they are growing and dividing more rapidly than most normal cells and cancer cells cannot repair the damage inflicted by chemotherapy as well as normal cells. However, some normal healthy cells that are growing and turning over rapidly are also affected by chemotherapy. These include **bone marrow** cells which make cells that clot blood, carry oxygen and fight infection. Other examples of cells that turn over rapidly include hair follicle lining cells and cells lining the gut. Therefore, some cytotoxic drugs can cause hair loss and digestive problems. Most normal tissues can

cytotoxic drugs
Drugs used as part of chemotherapy to kill cancer cells.

bone marrow
Blood-making cells situated in bones.

repair themselves and fully recover after chemotherapy has been completed.

There are over 50 types of cytotoxic drug and many are used in the treatment of lung cancer. Most cytotoxic drugs are given intravenously by drip or injection through a cannula in the arm (see Figure 6.1) although some can be given by mouth in tablet form. Different drugs are combined to make up chemotherapy regimes which are used to treat specific types of cancers including lung cancer.

Chemotherapy is usually given at intervals of three to four weeks and this is known as a cycle of chemotherapy. A course of chemotherapy is made up of a number of cycles; typically a course of chemotherapy will consist of three to six cycles depending on the reason for giving it.

Q How is the dose of chemotherapy calculated?

A It is usually based on a patient's height and weight. There can be other methods used for certain drugs such as using kidney function to work out the dose of drug. Modifications are sometimes required if the side-effects are too severe.

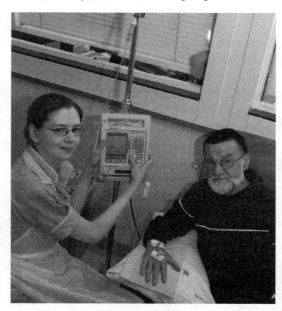

Fig 6.1 A patient receiving intravenous chemotherapy for lung cancer.

Side-effects

Virtually all chemotherapy drugs or combinations of drugs will have side-effects but these will vary greatly from person to person and most side-effects can be effectively treated. Some side-effects are common to most chemotherapy drugs and some are specific to the drug concerned. General side-effects which are common to most cytotoxic drugs are listed below; side-effects which are more specific are discussed under the drug concerned.

> **my experience**
>
> My oncologist told me I had to have chemotherapy as my lung cancer had spread to my liver. I was very anxious because a friend who had had chemotherapy a few years ago had a very bad time with it. I was given information about what to expect from chemotherapy and was pleasantly surprised to find that I had very few side-effects. Those that I did experience only lasted for a few days in the three week cycle and my symptoms improved during the chemotherapy.

Bone marrow suppression

The bone marrow produces the different cells which circulate in the blood. The three main types of cells produced in the bone marrow are:

- ✧ red blood cells which contain **haemoglobin** and carry oxygen around the body
- ✧ white blood cells which make up part of the immune system and fight infection
- ✧ platelets that help the blood to clot.

Bone marrow is very active, with blood cells being produced all the time, so chemotherapy which affects rapidly growing cells can temporarily affect and slow down the production of these

haemoglobin
An iron-containing protein which carries oxygen around the body to tissues.

cells leading to side-effects. Chemotherapy can affect the bone marrow at any time but the most common time is about ten to 14 days into each cycle of chemotherapy.

Red blood cells

Chemotherapy can lead to a reduction in the number of red blood cells, causing symptoms of anaemia which include tiredness, lethargy, weakness and breathlessness. Blood transfusions or drugs, such as **erythropoietin**, can be given to make the bone marrow work better. Anaemia can sometimes be cumulative, with symptoms getting worse as the chemotherapy progresses.

erythropoietin

A naturally occurring protein which stimulates bone marrow to make red blood cells. It can be given as a drug by injection under the skin to help treat anaemia related to chemotherapy.

White blood cells

A reduction in the number of white blood cells can make patients more prone to infections. Usually the numbers of white cells recover by the time the next cycle of chemotherapy is due. **Neutrophils** are a special type of white blood cell that are especially important in fighting infections, therefore it is particularly important that the number of neutrophils has recovered before the next cycle of chemotherapy is given. Symptoms of an infection can include a high temperature (above 38 °C), shivering or shaking (rigors), or suddenly feeling unwell. If this occurs then patients need to contact their oncology department promptly. Outside normal working hours patients will be given a specific telephone number to contact for help and advice as they may have a severe infection and may need to be admitted to hospital for antibiotic treatment. Oral antibiotics may be given for part of the

neutrophils

A type of white blood cell which help the body fight infection. (Also known as, granulocytes.)

chemotherapy cycle to reduce the chances of a severe infection. Occasionally growth factors such as granulocyte colony stimulating factor (**GCSF**) are given during chemotherapy or with a severe infection to help the white cells recover more quickly.

GCSF
A naturally occurring protein which can be given as a drug by injection to stimulate the production of white cells.

Platelets

A low platelet count increases the risk of bruising and unexpected bleeding. If this happens the patient needs to contact their oncology department promptly as they may need a transfusion of platelets. However, this is quite rare. Like white blood cells, platelets recover after a few days, usually in time for the next chemotherapy cycle.

myth
Patients having chemotherapy must stay away from public places in case they pick up infections.

fact
An infection can be picked up anywhere. Patients do not need to isolate themselves from others.

Nausea and vomiting

Many people who are to have chemotherapy are worried about nausea and vomiting. Although this can be a side-effect of chemotherapy it can be prevented or controlled with anti-sickness (anti-emetic) medication. These drugs may be given before and after chemotherapy, by tablet, injection or suppository. If symptoms of nausea or vomiting develop or persist patients should contact their doctor or nurse as other medicines can be prescribed.

myth
Everyone who has chemotherapy suffers from nausea or vomiting.

fact
Although this is a common side-effect many people do not suffer from this, especially with the chemotherapy combinations in current use for lung cancer. Drugs given to prevent nausea and sickness are usually very effective.

Loss of appetite

This may occur even if nausea and vomiting are controlled. It may result from abnormal taste sensations as a result of the chemotherapy. If it is severe then a dietician should be consulted.

Hair loss

Hair loss can be a problem with some drugs but it is not universal so it is important to find out whether a particular drug or combination may cause this problem. Hair loss usually starts two to three weeks after commencing chemotherapy and lasts for the duration of the treatment. Hair starts to grow back again a few months after treatment has been completed. Oncologists and chemotherapy nurses can give advice on hair loss and how best to cope with it.

Fertility and contraception

Chemotherapy drugs can affect both female and male fertility. If this is relevant then it should be discussed with the patient and his or her partner before starting chemotherapy. Chemotherapy drugs could potentially harm a foetus so it is very important not to become pregnant or father a child during chemotherapy. Although chemotherapy can affect fertility it is important to take proper contraceptive measures during treatment.

How is chemotherapy given?

Cytotoxic chemotherapy is usually given intravenously. In most cases treatment is supervised by an oncologist and administered by a specially trained chemotherapy nurse.

Q **Can I work between chemotherapy sessions?**

A This very much depends on the nature of your job, how you are feeling generally and what side-effects you experience. If you are feeling well there is no reason why you should not work but there may well be days when you feel less well and should not work. It is important to discuss this with your oncologist and also your employer who should understand why you may not be able to work normally. If your job is very demanding then it is advisable to try to reduce the intensity of work or the hours worked.

Patients are seen in an out-patient clinic prior to chemotherapy. If they have experienced specific side-effects with previous cycles of treatment the doctors and nurses treating them may be able to modify the treatment or give medications to help counter side-effects. It is important that it is safe to administer chemotherapy so blood tests which monitor bone marrow, kidney and liver function are taken and checked before going ahead with a

Q **Can I drive whilst I am having chemotherapy?**

A It is safe to drive but it is recommended that immediately after chemotherapy is given a friend or relative should drive the patient home, particularly after the first cycle, in case there are side-effects.

cycle of chemotherapy. Chemotherapy regimes differ in the time taken to give them and some can be administered in less than an hour whilst some will take all day to give and may need admission to hospital for the day or an overnight stay.

When blood tests have established it is safe to go ahead with a cycle of chemotherapy the chemotherapy nurse will insert a cannula into a vein, usually in a patient's forearm, and administer the chemotherapy. Cytotoxic drugs can irritate veins so, when the drug is being administered, a close check is kept on the vein. If access to veins is poor then there are alternative ways of getting the chemotherapy into a vein. This is usually with a specially inserted tube into a larger neck or arm vein which remains in place in between cycles of chemotherapy.

my experience

After two or three chemotherapy sessions the chemotherapy nurses had great difficulty in finding a suitable vein for my chemotherapy. They suggested a special line which is tunnelled under the skin and goes into a large vein in my chest. I had this put in under sedation and now I don't need to worry about them finding veins anymore. They can also take blood from it for tests. The district nurse helps me look after it.

When is chemotherapy given?

There are various indications for chemotherapy in the treatment of both NSCLC and small cell lung cancer. As with radiotherapy, factors such as the stage of the tumour and the general fitness and health of the patient will determine whether chemotherapy is appropriate and which type should be given.

Treatment for non-small cell lung cancer (NSCLC)

Neo-adjuvant chemotherapy

Chemotherapy can be given prior to surgery when a tumour is operable, although this is rarely done. This is called neo-adjuvant chemotherapy. Reasons for doing this include: treatment of **micro-metastatic disease**; trying to reduce the size or extent of the tumour to make the operation easier, or it may be easier to give the chemotherapy before surgery rather than after it.

Even if a tumour is operable there may be microscopic deposits of cancer present elsewhere in the body – too small to be detected by scans or blood tests – and chemotherapy may kill these deposits before they grow. If a tumour can only be removed by taking out the whole lung (pneumonectomy) chemotherapy may reduce the size of the tumour such that it is only necessary to remove a lobe of lung (lobectomy). After surgery a patient may need a prolonged period of recovery and might not be able to tolerate adjuvant chemotherapy.

A possible disadvantage of this treatment is that it delays surgery and theoretically the tumour could grow. Neo-adjuvant chemotherapy is still under evaluation and the results of clinical trials are awaited. Usually two or three cycles of chemotherapy are given.

Down-staging chemotherapy

This is similar to neo-adjuvant chemotherapy in that treatment is given prior to surgery. In this situation, however, the tumour is not operable before chemotherapy is given and the treatment

> **micro-metastatic disease**
> Disease which has spread in an amount so small it cannot be seen by conventional scans or blood tests.

Q How do doctors decide who can have down-staging chemotherapy?

A Doctors should discuss all new cases of lung cancer in a multi-disciplinary meeting. If it is felt that a tumour is in a location where surgery may be possible and if it can be shrunk down then they may recommend down-staging chemotherapy.

is designed to shrink the tumour or associated lymph nodes in the mediastinum. In order to assess whether this has been successful further tests may be necessary prior to surgery. Two to three cycles of chemotherapy are given.

Adjuvant chemotherapy

Chemotherapy can be given following surgery as an 'insurance policy' to reduce the risk of the cancer returning. This is called adjuvant chemotherapy. Recent clinical trials have shown that this treatment is of benefit following surgical resection of a lung cancer. The results suggest that there may be an improvement in survival following surgery of up to ten per cent when adjuvant chemotherapy is given.

Chemotherapy should start soon after surgery when the patient has made a good recovery – probably after four to eight weeks. Up to four cycles of chemotherapy are recommended. If there is evidence of a tumour having been left behind, chemotherapy may be scheduled either before or after post-operative radiotherapy.

my experience After my operation an appointment was made for me to see an oncologist. He explained that my tumour had been completely removed and that one of the lymph nodes in my chest had also been removed because it contained a tumour. It was a Stage T2N1 tumour. He explained that it has been shown by research that giving chemotherapy reduces the chance of the cancer returning by about ten per cent. I did not expect to be offered chemotherapy and I wasn't sure I wanted it after such a big operation. The lung cancer nurse gave me some written information about the chemotherapy and I am currently discussing whether I am going to have it with my family.

Chemo-radiotherapy

Chemotherapy can be combined with radiotherapy to try to improve the results of radiotherapy alone. The main methods of combining the treatments are:

✧ sequential chemoradiotherapy – where chemotherapy is given first and then followed by radiotherapy

✧ concurrent chemoradiotherapy – when the treatments are given at the same time

When treatment is given sequentially full doses of chemotherapy can be given and the respective side-effects of chemotherapy and radiotherapy are separated. Two to four cycles of chemotherapy are given prior to radiotherapy. When chemotherapy is given concurrently the dose of chemotherapy may be reduced to lessen the toxicity of the combined treatments. Chemotherapy drugs can make cells more sensitive to radiation and, in order to optimize this, chemotherapy can be given in smaller doses on a daily or weekly basis with the radiotherapy. Adding chemotherapy to radiotherapy seems to improve the survival rates of radiotherapy alone by around five per cent, but increased side-effects are associated with concurrent treatment. Chemo-radiotherapy in one form or another is indicated for Stage 3A and some types of Stage 3B disease.

Palliative chemotherapy

Chemotherapy for Stage 3B or 4 disease is aimed at helping to alleviate symptoms when the disease cannot be cured. Chemotherapy has

Q What does a ten per cent improvement in survival mean?

A If after surgery statistics show that about 50 per cent of people are alive five years after their operation, a treatment which improves survival by ten per cent means that on average 60 per cent of people will be alive after five years. It is an average figure based on what has happened to a large number of people who have been in this situation. It is difficult to apply it to one individual.

been shown to improve symptoms, improve quality of life and prolong survival in this situation; but it is important to monitor treatment closely to make sure the treatment is of benefit to the individual patient.

The most important factor in assessing whether chemotherapy is going to be helpful is to assess the general level of fitness of a patient. This measurement is known as the performance status. A performance status of 0 means that a patient is fully active; a score of 1 means that they may need some assistance or they may feel a little tired and lethargic but are still able to carry out light tasks; a score of 2 indicates that they are able to walk and are capable of caring for themselves but are unable to carry out work activities; a score of 3 means that they are only capable of limited self-care and they are confined to a bed or chair for 50 per cent of their waking hours; finally, a score of 4 indicates that they are completely disabled and require complete and total nursing care (see Chapter 1, Figure 1.9). Patients with a good performance score of 0 or 1 are usually able to tolerate chemotherapy and most importantly gain benefit from it, whereas those with a higher score are unlikely to do so.

It is important to explain to patients who are about to undergo palliative chemotherapy and who have symptoms that they should start to feel the benefit during treatment, usually after one or two cycles. If they are not improving or getting a lot of toxicity or side-effects their oncologist should consider stopping the treatment or changing it.

Clinical trials have shown that there is no one chemotherapy regime which is clearly better than all the others, so the potential side-effects of a regime are important. Research has also shown that on average chemotherapy will improve survival by a few months and increases the chance of a patient being alive one year after diagnosis. It is essential to explain that these figures represent an average and that many people will fair better (or worse) than average, so close monitoring and discussion is required of anyone having chemotherapy in this situation.

On average four cycles of chemotherapy are given in advanced or metastatic disease. If an individual is responding well there may be a case to carry on to six cycles but, equally, if they are not responding they may wish to stop after one or two cycles as further cycles are unlikely to be of benefit.

myth
Everyone needs to have six cycles of chemotherapy.

fact
Patients having palliative chemotherapy for lung cancer need to be assessed frequently to make sure they are responding to treatment and are not experiencing too many side-effects. Responding to treatment may mean that the cancer is getting smaller on a scan or X-ray or that symptoms are improving even when no major changes can be seen on scans. Many people will not have as many as six cycles – sometimes the maximum benefit from chemotherapy is seen after three or four cycles of treatment. If chemotherapy does not improve symptoms after one or two cycles or has a lot of side-effects it may be stopped and alternative treatments suggested.

Second line chemotherapy

If a lung cancer returns or grows again chemotherapy can sometimes be repeated. The drugs used tend to be different as the cancer cells which remain are likely to be resistant to the original chemotherapy regime. The side-effects experienced may be different but it is still essential to monitor the treatment closely to make sure it is of benefit.

my experience

Six months after I completed chemotherapy I felt unwell and a scan showed that my lung cancer had returned. My oncologist offered me more chemotherapy of a different sort. This time round the treatment was a bit tougher and I had three cycles. My scan shows that the cancer is a little smaller and I feel that my symptoms have improved.

Treatment for small cell lung cancer (SCLC)

Limited stage disease

In around one-third of small cell lung cancer the disease is classified as limited stage disease (see p. 25). It may, therefore, be possible to contain the disease or in a few cases cure the cancer with aggressive treatment. The most common treatment in this situation is a combination of chemotherapy and radiotherapy. Chemotherapy is chosen because small cell lung cancer tends to spread to other areas of the body and as chemotherapy is a systemic whole body treatment it will treat all areas. Small cell lung cancer is also very sensitive to chemotherapy and will respond to treatment in around 70–80 per cent of cases. If the tumour responds well to chemotherapy, radiotherapy is usually added to the treatment as this has been shown to improve results. Radiotherapy may be given during or sometimes after the chemotherapy. In limited stage disease up to six cycles are given depending on how the tumour is responding.

Q Can small cell lung cancer be cured?

A Treatment can be curative in limited stage small cell lung cancer. However, the cancer does have a tendency to return, usually within the first two years. A small percentage of limited stage small cell lung cancer (less than 20 per cent) can be cured with a combination of chemotherapy and radiotherapy.

Extensive stage disease

In around two-thirds of cases of small cell lung cancer tests show that the cancer has spread from the chest or thorax to other areas. Parts of the body where small cell lung cancer commonly spreads to include the liver, bones, brain and adrenal glands. When this happens it is not possible to eradicate the disease completely but it is possible to control it and help symptoms associated with it. The main treatment for extensive stage small cell lung cancer is chemotherapy. Small cell lung cancer is very sensitive to chemotherapy and likely to respond to treatment, but in extensive stage disease the cancer tends to return at a later stage.

Chemotherapy has been shown to improve symptoms, improve quality of life and prolong survival in this situation, but it is important to monitor treatment closely to make sure the treatment is of benefit to the individual patient. The most important factor in assessing whether chemotherapy is going to be helpful is to assess the general level of fitness of a patient. This is a measurement known as the performance status (see Chapter 1, Figure 1.9).

As mentioned earlier, it is important that the medical team explains to the patient that they should start to feel the benefit during treatment, usually after one or two cycles. If they are not improving or getting a lot of toxicity or side-effects their oncologist should consider stopping the treatment or changing it. Most people with extensive stage small cell lung cancer who are having chemotherapy and are responding well have between four and six cycles.

 How can quality of life be measured?

 This can be done by simply asking someone whether their symptoms are changing for better or worse, or it can be measured by asking specific questions in a questionnaire and scoring symptoms.

my experience

My doctor recommended that I have chemotherapy for small cell lung cancer which had spread to my lymph glands and bones. At first the chemotherapy helped my cough but after three cycles I felt exhausted and I could not go on with the treatment. I explained this to the doctor and he felt that I had got as much benefit as I was going to get and stopped the treatment. After a week or two I felt much better and I am now enjoying life. I feel this is an important time for me and my family and I am aware that the cancer is likely to return.

Adjuvant chemotherapy

In very rare circumstances it may be possible to remove a small cell lung cancer surgically. In this situation post-operative or adjuvant chemotherapy is usually recommended. The reason for this is that small cell lung cancer can spread readily to other areas of the body and this may be too small to be seen by conventional scans or blood tests. Adjuvant chemotherapy is given as an 'insurance policy' to reduce the chance of the cancer recurring.

Chemotherapy regimens

A lot of people are very frightened when chemotherapy is recommended as part of their treatment. They are usually worried that they will feel very unwell during their treatment or that they will have have a lot of side-effects. It is important that the medical and nursing team who are looking after the patient explains what is involved in having chemotherapy and what side-effects to expect. The severity of side-effects will vary from person to person and the side-effects of chemotherapy regimens are not all the same. Patients may have heard of the experiences of others who have had different sorts of chemotherapy for different types of cancer. Everyone has a different experience and while it is important to inform people of potential side-effects it is essential to stress that most people will experience only a few of the side-effects discussed with them.

Most chemotherapy for both small cell and non-small cell lung cancer is given as a combination of cytotoxic drugs. A platinum-containing drug (cisplatin or carboplatin) is commonly used in combination with one or two other drugs. There are many different effective combinations of drugs. There are a number of different factors that your oncologist will take into account when deciding which treatment to offer you. They will be able to explain to you which combination of drugs is best suited to you and your lung cancer and why. Descriptions of the different types of drugs frequently used to treat lung cancer are listed on the following pages.

When chemotherapy is given for the first time in the treatment of lung cancer it is sometimes referred to as 'first line' chemotherapy. If the lung cancer returns following treatment or is not responding to the initial treatment a 'second line' chemotherapy regimen may be used. Usually a different type of cytotoxic drug or drugs will be used in this situation as it is felt that the cancer is now resistant to the chemotherapy regimen which was used as first line treatment.

Chemotherapy drugs

Carboplatin

Carboplatin is another platinum-containing drug. It is given as an intravenous infusion via a drip and normally takes around 30 minutes to give. The dose of carboplatin is usually worked out from a patient's kidney function rather than their

GFR

This stands for Glomerular Filtration Rate. A measurement of how well the kidneys are working.

Q How do doctors work out the dose of chemotherapy to give to a patient?

A This is based on a patient's height, weight and possibly other factors such as their general health or kidney function. In certain situations the dose of chemotherapy may need to be adjusted depending on how the first cycle is tolerated.

height and weight. Patients may be asked to attend for a special kidney test (**GFR**) or to collect their urine over a 24-hour period before chemotherapy starts. The main side-effect of carboplatin is:

✧ Temporary bone marrow damage – carboplatin most commonly affects the bone marrow cells which produce platelets which help the blood to clot. If bruising or bleeding problems are noticed then this should be reported immediately to the oncology team. Carboplatin can also affect the bone marrow cells which produce red and white blood cells, so symptoms of anaemia, such as tiredness and a raised temperature associated with infection, need to be looked for.

Less common side-effects with carboplatin can include:

✧ Nausea and vomiting – which can be controlled with anti-sickness medication.
✧ Tingling in the hands and feet or hearing problems – this can be due to nerve damage and is cumulative so should be reported to the oncologist if experienced.
✧ Allergic reaction – feeling unwell immediately after or during the second or subsequent cycle. This needs to be reported to the nurse or oncologist as the chemotherapy may need to be altered.

Cisplatin

Cisplatin is a clear fluid which is given intravenously via a drip, usually on the first day of

a three or four week chemotherapy cycle.
Cisplatin is usually given with other intravenous
fluid and typically takes six to eight hours to give.
The main side-effects of cisplatin are:

✧ Nausea and vomiting – this can occur a few
hours or days after the drug has been given.
It can be prevented by giving anti-emetics
(anti-sickness) medication before and after
chemotherapy has been given. If it does
develop or persist other anti-sickness
medication can be effective in controlling
this problem.

✧ Kidney damage – cisplatin can damage
renal (kidney) function, especially if the
kidneys are not working normally. Cisplatin
is given with a lot of intravenous fluid (pre-
hydration and post-hydration) which is
supplemented with **magnesium and
potassium salts** to prevent this kidney
damage. It is also important to check renal
function before starting cisplatin-based
chemotherapy and to monitor it during
cycles of treatment. The easiest way of
doing this is to monitor the level of
creatinine in the blood – a raised level
indicates reduced kidney function.

✧ Temporary bone marrow damage – cisplatin
like most cytotoxic drugs can affect the
production of blood cells in the bone
marrow. It most commonly affects the red
blood cells which carry oxygen around the
body; if you are found to be anaemic during
chemotherapy you may be offered
treatment to correct this (a blood transfusion
or erythropoietin injections). Cisplatin can
also affect other parts of the bone marrow

**magnesium and
potassium salts**
Chemicals which
occur naturally in the
body and which are
essential for
metabolism.

creatinine
A natural by-product of
metabolism that is
excreted by the kidneys.

which produce the white blood cells and the platelets. These white blood cells fight infection and the platelets help the blood to clot.

Less common side-effects can include:

tinnitus
Ringing in the ears.

✧ Changes in hearing – cisplatin can sometimes cause **tinnitus** or high tone hearing loss. If this is noticed it should be reported to the doctor as further tests or alterations to the dose of drug may need to be made.

✧ Taste changes – some people notice an alteration to their taste – either a metallic taste or food becomes less appetizing. It is usually temporary.

✧ Nerve damage – cisplatin can cause a tingling sensation in the hands and feet (peripheral neuropathy). This can be uncomfortable and cumulative so it is important that if it is experienced it is reported to a doctor or chemotherapy nurse.

Cyclophosphamide

Cyclophosphamide is given as an intravenous injection or infusion over a few minutes. Side-effects can include:

✧ nausea and vomiting
✧ risk of infection and bleeding
✧ tiredness
✧ hair loss
✧ irritation of the bladder lining which may give symptoms of cystitis
✧ a very rare risk of second cancers forming many years later.

Docetaxel

Docetaxel is given by intravenous infusion. It takes around one hour to give and is usually given on the first day of the chemotherapy cycle with cisplatin or carboplatin but can also be given on its own as second line chemotherapy if the cancer has returned. Docetaxel is given in conjunction with a short course of steroid tablets or an injection (dexamethasone) just before and after the infusion to prevent allergic reactions to the treatment. Side-effects can include:

✧ nausea and vomiting – usually mild
✧ risk of infection and bleeding
✧ tiredness
✧ changes to skin and nails
✧ allergic reaction
✧ fluid retention
✧ tingling in the hands and feet
✧ sore mouth
✧ hair loss.

Doxorubicin

Doxorubicin is a red-coloured drug which is given by intravenous injection into the vein over a few minutes. Side-effects can include:

✧ nausea and vomiting
✧ risk of infection and bleeding
✧ tiredness
✧ hair loss
✧ heart damage if given in high doses
✧ red discolouration of urine
✧ irritation to the veins and if the drug leaks out of a vein it can cause damage to the surrounding tissue. When the drug is given

the chemotherapy nurse will check for this very carefully
✧ sore mouth or mouth ulcers.

Etoposide

Etoposide is given by intravenous infusion over one hour or in oral capsule form. It is usually given on the first few days of the chemotherapy cycle. It is sometimes given intravenously on the first and possibly second day and orally on the next few days. Side-effects can include:

✧ nausea and vomiting
✧ risk of infection and bleeding
✧ tiredness
✧ hair loss
✧ diahorrea
✧ sore mouth
✧ a very rare risk of second cancers forming many years later.

Gemcitabine

Gemcitabine is given by a short intravenous infusion into a vein, which takes around 15–20 minutes. It is usually given on the first day of a chemotherapy cycle with a platinum-containing drug and may also be given on its own in the second week of the three-week chemotherapy cycle. Side-effects can include:

✧ nausea and vomiting – usually mild
✧ risk of infection and bleeding
✧ tiredness
✧ drowsiness
✧ temporary increase in breathlessness
✧ rash.

Q **What is an intravenous infusion?**

A Sometimes a drug can be injected into a vein using a needle and syringe. This is an intravenous injection. However, sometimes a drug is put in a small bag of saline and allowed to trickle into a vein as a drip. This is called an intravenous infusion. The method by which your treatment is given depends upon the drug. Your oncology doctor or the lung cancer nurse specialist will explain which drugs you are to have, how they will be given and how long this treatement will take.

Ifosfamide

Ifosfamide is given as an intravenous infusion over a few hours. Side-effects can include:

✧ nausea and vomiting
✧ risk of infection and bleeding
✧ tiredness
✧ hair loss
✧ irritation of the bladder lining which may give symptoms of cystitis. It is usually given with another drug called mesna to counteract this.

Paclitaxel

Paclitaxel is given by intravenous infusion. It takes a few hours to give and is usually given on the first day of the chemotherapy cycle with cisplatin or carboplatin. Paclitaxel may be given with pre-medication of steroids and anti-stomach acid medications. Paclitaxel and docetaxel are members of the same family of chemotherapy drugs – taxanes. Side-effects can include:

✧ nausea and vomiting – usually mild
✧ risk of infection and bleeding

✧ tiredness
✧ changes to skin
✧ allergic reaction
✧ tingling in the hands and feet
✧ sore mouth
✧ hair loss.

Pemetrexed

Pemetrexed is given by a short intravenous infusion which takes about ten to 15 minutes. Before starting chemotherapy with pemetrexed, patients are pre-medicated with folic acid tablets and vitamin B12 injections one to two weeks before chemotherapy starts. Folic acid is then taken daily during treatment and for three weeks afterwards and vitamin B12 injections are given every eight to nine weeks during treatment. Steroid tablets (dexamethasone) are also given just before chemotherapy to prevent an allergic rash. Side-effects can include:

✧ nausea and vomiting – usually mild
✧ risk of infection and bleeding
✧ tiredness
✧ rash.

Vinblastine and Mitomycin C

Vinblastine and mitomycin C are given by intravenous infusion on the first day of a chemotherapy cycle. Sometimes mitomycin C is given only every other cycle. They only take a few minutes to give. Side-effects can include:

✧ nausea and vomiting – usually mild
✧ risk of infection and bleeding
✧ tiredness
✧ constipation

✧ tingling in the hands and feet
✧ irritation to the veins and if the drug leaks out of a vein it can cause damage to the surrounding tissue. When the drug is given the chemotherapy nurse will observe for this very closely.

Vincristine

Vincristine is given as an injection into the vein over a few minutes. Side-effects can include:

✧ nausea and vomiting – usually mild
✧ risk of infection and bleeding
✧ tiredness
✧ constipation
✧ tingling in the hands and feet
✧ irritation to the veins and if the drug leaks out of a vein it can cause damage to the surrounding tissue. When the drug is given the chemotherapy nurse will observe for this very closely.

Vinorelbine

Vinorelbine is given by an intravenous injection into the vein which takes around ten minutes. It is also available as an oral medication taken as a capsule. It is usually given on the first day of a chemotherapy cycle with a platinum-containing drug and may also be given on its own in the second week of the three-week chemotherapy cycle. If given as a capsule it is also given on the first day of the cycle and one week later. Side-effects can include:

✧ nausea and vomiting – usually mild
✧ risk of infection and bleeding

✧ tiredness
✧ constipation, although the capsule form can also cause diarrhoea
✧ tingling in the hands and feet
✧ irritation to the veins if given intravenously and if the drug leaks out of a vein it can cause damage to the surrounding tissue. When the drug is given the chemotherapy nurse will observe for this very closely.

CHAPTER

7

Other treatments

In this chapter we describe a number of other treatments for lung cancer that your lung cancer specialist may discuss with you depending upon your particular circumstances and needs. A number of the treatments are specialized and are not available in every hospital. In some cases you may have to visit a specialist centre to be treated. Your doctors will advise you about whether these treatments will help you.

Growth factor inhibitors

Growth factor inhibitors are a new type of drug for treating cancers. **Growth factors** are molecules present in the body which cause cells to grow and divide. Cancer cells, like normal cells, respond to growth factors and multiply. However, unlike normal cells, cancer cells often grow faster and in a disorganized fashion. Growth factors stimulate cells by attaching to

growth factors
Substances which circulate in the body and have an effect on cells, usually by attaching to receptors and causing cells to become more active.

receptor
A protein on the surface of a cell which acts as a switch for activities within the cell.

monoclonal antibodies
Special proteins which recognize a particular receptor on a cell surface.

enzymes
Proteins which help biological reactions take place.

special **receptors** on the surface of the cell and causing signals to be passed to the nucleus of the cell telling them to grow. Growth factor inhibitors work by blocking these receptors and therefore preventing the growth signals from occurring. At present scientists are trying to develop different types of drugs to block growth signals. One type is called **monoclonal antibodies**, which attach to growth factor receptors on cancer cells and block them from working. Another group of drugs under development are designed to block the **enzyme** signals that pass the signals from the growth factor receptors to the nucleus of the cell. At present, there are a number of drugs in both groups undergoing clinical trials. Some may enter routine clinical use in the future. One type of drug, called an epidermal growth factor receptor inhibitor, has already been shown to work in lung cancer and has entered clinical practice.

Epidermal growth factor receptor (EGFR) inhibitors

Some types of lung cancer cells have a special type of growth factor receptor on their surface called an epidermal growth factor receptor. Epidermal growth factor receptor inhibitors are a new type of drug that has been found to attach to the epidermal growth factor receptor and prevent it sending growth signals to the nucleus of the cell. The drug (erlotinib or Tarceva®) blocks a specific enzyme called tyrosine kinase from sending out a signal to the nucleus. It is given in tablet form and tablets are taken once a day. It is taken for as long as it is seen to be giving benefit. Recent research has shown that erlotinib can shrink down tumours in a small number of cases but it may also work by stopping cancer cells growing rather than killing them outright and so stabilizing the disease.

Side-effects are generally not as severe as chemotherapy but can include:

✧ a rash, which starts after a week or two. It can resemble acne and affect the face and other parts of the body
✧ diarrhoea, which is usually quite mild and does not need any special treatment
✧ fatigue or tiredness
✧ a sore mouth
✧ nausea or vomiting in rare cases.

At present erlotinib is used to treat patients with lung cancer that has returned after initial standard chemotherapy. Research is currently underway to find out whether erlotinib can be used instead of chemotherapy when people are too frail to receive chemotherapy. It is already known that erlotinib is not effective if given together with chemotherapy. Work is also underway to see if there are any tests that can be done on a particular individual's cancer to see if it more likely to respond to erlotinib. At present there are no tests which can reliably do this. It has been observed that some people may benefit more than others from erlotinib. These include people who have never smoked, women, people with adenocarcinoma and those of south-east Asian origin. However, this does not mean that other people may not benefit from erlotinib.

Q **Since I started erlotinib I have come out in a rash. How can I best deal with this?**

A There is no single treatment – using a moisturizer may help and some masking creams can be used to cover up the rash. Anti-acne treatments are not recommended.

Q **When do paraneoplastic syndromes occur?**

A There is no particular reason why paraneoplastic syndromes occur but they tend to occur in certain types of cancer. Hypercalcaemia usually occurs when a lung cancer is of the squamous cell type. Paraneoplastic syndromes are more common in small cell lung cancer.

my experience

A few months after I completed my chemotherapy my cough came back, I was getting more breathless and tests showed that my cancer was returning. My oncologist suggested more chemotherapy but I just couldn't face it so he prescribed erlotinib. I have been on the tablets for six weeks now and my breathlessness is a little better and my X-ray is stable. I think that the erlotinib tablets have stopped my disease from getting worse. Unlike chemotherapy I have few side-effects and I can stay on the tablets for as long as they are holding the lung cancer in check.

How to treat hypercalcaemia

Hypercalcaemia can be a problem in lung cancer when cancer spreads to the bones and releases too much calcium into the blood. It can also be seen when the primary cancer in the lung produces a substance (hormone) which causes calcium to be released from the bones without spreading directly to the bones themselves. This is called a paraneoplastic syndrome.

hypercalcaemia
Elevated calcium levels in the blood.

Symptoms of **hypercalcaemia** can include abdominal pain, constipation, confusion and thirst. It is diagnosed by a blood test. The treatment of hypercalceamia is to give lots of fluids, usually intravenously, to flush away the high calcium content and then to treat with intravenous bisphosphonates.

Using bisphosphonates to treat secondary bone cancer

Secondary bone cancer can present with symptoms of pain in the bones, or a fracture of a bone, as well as hypercalcaemia.

Bisphosphonates are a group of drugs which can be used to treat high levels of calcium in the body (hypercalceamia) and also to treat bones that have been affected by lung cancer metastasis (secondary bone cancer).

Bisphosphonates can be given either in tablet form or via an intravenous infusion. The most common types of bisphosphonates used when lung cancer has spread to bones or is causing hypercalcaemia are pamidronate or zolendronic acid. These drugs are given by intravenous infusion into a vein over a period of 15–90 minutes depending on which drug is being used. Side-effects of bisphosphonates are:

✧ high temperature and flu-like symptoms or chills for a day or so after the infusion. This may be worse after the first infusion and be less of a problem for subsequent infusions
✧ aching in joints and muscles
✧ change in kidney function – your kidney function should be measured by blood tests.

Bisphosphonates given for hypercalcaemia are usually given as a one-off treatment but repeated if calcium levels rise again. Bisphosphonate infusions for bone pain are usually repeated every four weeks for as long as they are giving benefit.

Radiotherapy to affected bones or surgical repair (fixation) of fractures caused by secondary bone cancer may also be recommended.

Treatment of pleural effusions

If lung cancer spreads to the pleural membranes lining the outside of the lung, fluid can accumulate between the parietal pleura and visceral pleura (see figure 1.3). The build up of fluid in the space between the membranes is called a pleural effusion and can cause breathlessness and discomfort as it compresses the lung.

myth
Bisphosphonates are a form of chemotherapy.

fact
Although these drugs can be given by intravenous drip they are not a form of chemotherapy as they do not kill cells but alter the way the body makes new bone.

Pleural aspiration

It is possible to help these symptoms by draining off some of the fluid. This can be done by inserting a small cannula into the pleura and draining off some of the fluid. More fluid can be removed if a special drain is inserted into the chest and left to drain off as much fluid as possible. It may be necessary to locate the exact position of the fluid by an ultrasound scan but sometimes the fluid is present in separate pockets so it is not always possible to drain off all the fluid.

Medical pleurodesis

If all the fluid can be drained away (there may be as much as a few litres present) it is sometimes possible to 'stick' the two sheets of pleura together and prevent the fluid reaccumulating. This is done by injecting a drug down the chest drain and leaving it in for a short time before removing the drain. Sterile talc can be used for this purpose. Pleurodesis can be uncomfortable when the drug is first injected so appropriate painkillers and local anaesthetic should be given.

my experience

Over a period of a few weeks I noticed that I was becoming more breathless, especially when going up hills or climbing stairs. I mentioned this to my doctor when I went to see him. He organized a chest X-ray and this showed fluid in the chest or a pleural effusion. I was admitted to hospital and had a tube called a chest drain inserted into my chest under local anaesthetic. Over three litres of fluid drained off over the next two days. My breathing improved dramatically. When an X-ray showed all the fluid had been removed the doctor injected a mixture of sterile talc down the chest drain. This was rather uncomfortable for around a day but I was given painkillers. The drain was removed and my breathing is now much better and the fluid now cannot re-accumulate.

Surgical pleurodesis

This same procedure can sometimes be done surgically. This involves a small operation (mini-thoracotomy) or key hole surgery (thoracoscopy). This allows better drainage of the fluid and talc can be inserted directly into the pleural cavity. However this can involve a longer stay in hospital.

Surgery for metastatic disease

Surgical operations can sometimes be helpful when lung cancer has spread to other areas and is causing specific problems.

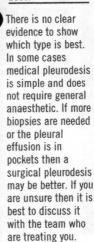

Q **Which type of pleurodesis is best?**

A There is no clear evidence to show which type is best. In some cases medical pleurodesis is simple and does not require general anaesthetic. If more biopsies are needed or the pleural effusion is in pockets then a surgical pleurodesis may be better. If you are unsure then it is best to discuss it with the team who are treating you.

Q **Why can't surgery be used to remove all metastatic disease?**

A Surgery is reserved for special situations because once a cancer has started to spread, as well as the disease that can been seen on scans, there is usually microscopic spread of the disease which cannot be seen. Surgery can only remove the disease that can be seen and will have no effect on the microscopic disease. Eventually the microscopic disease will grow. Sometimes the disease has spread to too many areas to remove it all or the metastasis is in a critical area that cannot be removed without causing major damage.

Brain metastasis

Neurosurgery can sometimes be helpful in special circumstances when lung cancer has spread to the brain. If there is evidence from CT and MRI scans that there is only one deposit of cancer in the brain, and if the lung cancer is under control elsewhere in the body, then an operation

Q **What are the signs and symptoms of lung cancer that has spread to the brain?**

A Signs and symptoms can include headaches which may be more severe in the morning, weakness of the arms and legs on one side, and difficulty with balance or dizziness. If brain metastases are suspected then usually a CT or MRI scan of the brain is needed to confirm this.

paraplegia
Weakness and sometimes loss of power of both legs caused by damage to the spinal cord.

to remove the metastasis may be possible. After neurosurgery a course of radiotherapy to the remainder of the brain is usually recommended. There are some parts of the brain where removal of a secondary deposit of cancer may be too dangerous. However it may be possible to treat these areas with stereotactic radiotherapy, sometimes known as gamma knife radiosurgery.

Spinal cord surgery

When lung cancer spreads to the bones of the spinal column or vertebrae it can occasionally press on the spinal cord running through the spinal column. This can affect the function of the spinal cord as pressure on it can cause numbness, weakness and paralysis (**paraplegia**) depending on the area of the spinal column affected.

The most common treatment for this condition is corticosteroid drugs (dexamethasone) and urgent radiotherapy. In special circumstances, if there is only one area of the spinal cord affected and if the disease is under control in the rest of the body and if the patient is not already weak or paralysed, then surgery to relieve the pressure from (decompress) the spinal cord might be recommended. After surgery post-operative radiotherapy is usually recommended.

Fixation of long bones

When lung cancer spreads to certain bones and causes them to fracture, surgery to re-join or fix them is recommended. Examples of this include the femur (thigh bone) and humerus (upper arm bone). A pin is usually inserted at operation by an orthopaedic surgeon and radiotherapy and possibly bisphosphonates are recommended after surgery.

Endobronchial treatments

In addition to palliative treatments such as chemotherapy and radiotherapy there are several **endobronchial treatments** that are sometimes used in conjunction with or instead of these treatments. Sometimes patients who are not fit enough for chemotherapy or radiotherapy or who have had the maximum doses of these treatments can have an endobronchial treatment in order to try to relieve symptoms. Endobronchial treatments can be useful for treating symptoms such as cough, breathlessness, haemoptysis, wheeze and repeated chest infections, all of which are being caused by a tumour within the airway.

At present the use of endobronchial treatments in the UK are limited to certain hospitals that specialize in the various techniques. It is likely that over the next few years these techniques will become more widespread.

endobronchial treatments
Techniques used to treat tumours that are positioned inside the airways.

 Q What is an endobronchial treatment?

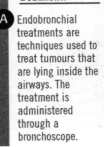 **A** Endobronchial treatments are techniques used to treat tumours that are lying inside the airways. The treatment is administered through a bronchoscope.

Endobronchial cryotherapy

Endobronchial cryotherapy or cryosurgery is a technique used to treat a tumour that is blocking or partially blocking an airway. It involves killing the tumour by freezing it inside the airway. During a bronchoscopy procedure (see Chapter 3) a thin probe is passed down through the bronchoscope until it touches the tumour. Using liquid nitrogen the tip of the probe is then cooled to about −70 °C which freezes the tumour around it. By repeated freeze-thaw cycles the tumour cells are killed and pieces of the dead tumour can be removed through the bronchoscope. The freezing of the tumour and its removal does not hurt. Quite often the cryotherapy treatment is repeated after a couple of weeks. The procedure can either be performed through a rigid bronchoscope under a general anaesthetic or through a flexible bronchoscope under sedation.

Endobronchial diathermy

Endobronchial diathermy or electrocautery is used for similar reasons as cryotherapy but involves cutting away the tumour tissue inside the airway using a high-temperature cutting probe. Like cryotherapy it can either be performed under a general anaesthetic or under sedation. Often the treatment can be delivered in just one session.

Endobronchial Nd:YAG laser therapy

This treatment involves using a laser to destroy tumour tissue inside the airway. A laser is an intense, narrow beam of light radiation. It transfers heat to the tumour tissue which results in cell death. The heat generated also destroys the blood vessels that supply the tumour. Again, this treatment can either be performed under a general anaesthetic or under sedation.

Endobronchial stents

Not all lung cancers occur inside the airways. Often they grow within the lung tissue adjacent to airways. As they enlarge, the tumour itself or the lymph glands containing the tumour can press on the airways and narrow them causing partial or

Q **What is a rigid bronchoscope?**

A A rigid bronchoscope is a hollow metal tube that can be inserted through the mouth and into the windpipe so that the inside of the lungs can be inspected and treated. The advantage of this technique over a flexible bronchoscope is that a rigid bronchoscope is much larger (up to one centimetre in diameter) and therefore this allows larger pieces of tumour tissue to be removed.

complete obstruction. This can cause symptoms of cough, breathlessness or repeated chest infections. In this situation a **stent** can be placed in the trachea or bronchial tubes to help keep the airway open. Stents are made of silicone, metal or a mesh material and can be placed in an airway before or after another treatment such as radiotherapy. Stents can either be placed through a rigid bronchoscope under general anaesthesia or through a flexible bronchoscope under sedation. X-ray screening is used to check the position of the stent before it is finally released. Often improvement in symptoms is immediate.

stent
An expandable hollow tube.

Photodynamic therapy (PDT)

Endobronchial photodynamic therapy combines a **photoactive drug** and light from a laser to kill cancer cells while limiting damage to surrounding healthy tissue. First of all a special drug called porfimer sodium is injected into a vein. The drug preferentially accumulates in cancer cells and sensitizes them to the effect of the laser light. Approximately 40–50 hours after the injection a bronchoscopy is performed and a low-power red light from a laser is shone onto the tumour tissue through a bronchoscope. The red light activates the porfimer sodium which destroys the cancer cells. A few days after the treatment another bronchoscopy is often performed to remove dead tumour tissue and mucus which has not been coughed up.

photoactive drug
A drug that is activated by light.

While this is a safe treatment it can have side-effects. Sometimes patients experience some chest or back discomfort as a result of local swelling and inflammation in the area around the tumour. In addition to accumulating in the tumour the drug accumulates in the skin. This means that the skin will be photosensitive for some time after the injection and exposure to sunlight can cause severe sunburn. Most of the effects will have worn off after four to six weeks but, occasionally, they may be more prolonged. Patients who have been injected with porfimer sodium have to ensure that they avoid direct sunlight during this time and this means staying indoors as much as possible. Normal indoor lighting is quite safe. If patients do go outdoors they are advised to cover all their skin and to wear a wide-brimmed hat and sunglasses.

Superior vena cava obstruction (SVCO) and treatments

The superior vena cava carries blood from the head and arms back to the heart. It can become blocked if a lung cancer presses against it or if lymph glands that lie next to the windpipe become enlarged. This can occur both in non-small cell lung cancer or small cell lung cancer although it is more common in the latter.

Patients will report symptoms of swelling in their neck, face or arms. They may complain of headache or a feeling of facial fullness and have a high colour. If the obstruction has been present for some time the blood may find alternative ways back to the heart by opening up smaller blood vessels across the front of the chest. There may be a bluish tinge to the skin in the upper half of the body. In order to relieve the blockage a stent can be inserted into the blood vessel to keep it open. The stent is usually inserted into a blood vessel in the groin and then pushed through the blood vessels of the abdomen until it is in the correct position inside the chest. The stent is guided into the correct position using X-ray screening. Use of a stent for this purpose normally gives rapid relief of symptoms. Prior to placement of a stent, high dose steroids (dexamethasone) may help symptoms in some patients.

If insertion of a stent is not possible then other treatments need to start as soon as possible. Treatment for SVCO will depend on the type of lung cancer but in many cases of small cell lung cancer chemotherapy will quickly relieve the obstruction. In non-small cell lung cancer a short course of palliative radiotherapy is usually recommended but chemotherapy may also be given.

Q What should I do if I think I have symptoms of spinal cord compression?

A If you think you have these symptoms then you should contact your GP or the team treating you straight away as urgent treatment may be required.

Spinal cord compression and treatments

When lung cancer spreads to the bones of the spinal column, it can cause pressure on the spinal cord or nerves coming from it. Symptoms of pain radiating down arms or legs, numbness, weakness, difficulty walking or difficulty passing urine can be experienced. If a spinal cord compression is suspected then the patient needs to be referred to hospital quickly in order for a diagnosis to be made. The need for diagnosis and treatment is urgent because, if left untreated, permanent nerve damage and paralysis can result. The best way of doing this is by MRI scanning of the spine which will clearly show if there is any tumour pressing on the spinal cord. Treatment often consists of high dose steroids and a short course of radiotherapy. In a few cases surgery, to decompress the spinal cord, may be performed.

Pericardial effusion and treatments

In some rare cases, lung cancer cells can spread to the sac that surrounds the heart (**pericardial sac**). This can cause fluid to build up within the sac (pericardial effusion), which in turn puts pressure on the heart.

pericardial sac
A sac of thin tissues which contains the heart.

If this occurs, the patient may have symptoms of breathlessness and a rapid heart rate. There may be swelling of veins in the neck. If a pericardial effusion is suspected, the patient must be referred to hospital urgently to have a heart scan (echocardiogram) performed. If this demonstrates fluid around the heart then it can be drained off by either inserting a small tube into the fluid guided by the echocardiogram (**pericardiocentesis**) or by an operation to open up a window in the pericardium allowing the fluid to drain off.

pericardiocentesis
Drainage of a pericardial effusion.

Clinical trials

oncology
The area of medicine that deals with the study and the treatment of cancer.

In all branches of **oncology**, doctors, nurses and other researchers are looking for new ways in which to improve cancer diagnosis and treatment. Patients may be asked to take part in trials or other forms of research. All forms of research will have been through a regulatory process to ensure the questions being asked are scientifically valid and ethical. Participation in a clinical trial or research is always voluntary and patients and their families should be given a description of the research in a language which they can understand and also be given time and information in a written form before making a decision about whether they wish to take part or not. There are many types of clinical trials.

Phase 1 trials

This is where a new drug or treatment is being tested for the first time in humans. The main aim of the trial is to see how safe it is and how much treatment can be given. Effects on the cancer will be noted but this is not the principal purpose of the trial.

Phase 2 trials

Lung cancer trials may be looking at a new treatment or method of diagnosing lung cancer. These trials look at how effective the treatment or test is, and this may be done before going on to compare it to the standard treatment or test.

Phase 3 trials

This is where there is a comparison with a standard method of treatment or diagnosis. Participation in such a trial may involve being randomly assigned to one type of treatment or investigation or another. This is known as a randomized controlled trial (RCT).

Blinded trials

In some clinical trials the patient and usually the doctors and nurses administering the treatment will be blinded to the treatment being given. This means that in order to avoid any bias, the

myth
Taking part in a clinical trial will mean that patients won't get properly treated.

fact
Patients should be reassured that if they take part in a clinical trial they will not go without treatment that their doctors feel they should definitely have. Some trials may involve a 'placebo' (dummy tablet or drug). If this is part of the trial it will mean that 'giving nothing' may be as good as the other treatment being investigated.

treatment is coded and it is not known whether the drug being given is the real drug being tested or a 'dummy' treatment (placebo). In emergency situations the clinical team treating the patient can 'break' the code and find out which treatment is being given. These trials are called blinded or double-blinded trials.

Before participating in any trial it is very important that the patient and their family fully understand why they are being asked to participate and what the trial involves.

Observational or non-interventional trials

These are not usually concerned with treatment but are trying to find out more about the condition or outcome of treatment. They may involve patients or their families filling in questionnaires about some aspect of their disease or treatment. It may involve giving a blood sample to see if more can be discovered about lung cancer.

All those taking part in clinical trials can ask to withdraw from a clinical trial at any time. They will not be penalized in any way. They should also feel free to ask questions at any time.

CHAPTER

8

Symptom control

Many lung cancer symptoms can be helped by treatments such as surgery, chemotherapy and radiotherapy. However, there are sometimes symptoms which do not respond to these treatments or persist after treatment has been given. Controlling these symptoms is important in all stages and types of lung cancer. Members of the specialist lung cancer team as well as doctors and nurses in the community will have expertise in treating such symptoms and so patients should feel confident about seeking help from them. The lung cancer specialist nurse is usually a good point of contact. He or she will be able to help or direct the patient to the person most able to help.

Common symptoms

Pain

Pain is a common symptom. There are many types of pain and a specialist may want to know more about the nature of the pain, in particular its frequency, severity, type and site. In order to help find the source of the pain more tests such as X-rays and scans may be ordered. There are a large number of painkillers (analgesics) available and different ones may be prescribed for different types of pain. Common side-effects of painkillers can include constipation and drowsiness and it is important to report these and any other side-effects as most can be dealt with. It may be possible to help relieve the pain with a nerve block and injections and these patients may need to be referred to a specialist pain clinic.

Radiotherapy and chemotherapy may also be useful in helping control pain by treating the tumour which is causing the pain.

Breathlessness

There are many reasons why someone with lung cancer can be breathless. The specialist team may need to do blood tests or X-rays and scans to determine the nature of the breathlessness. Common causes of breathlessness in lung cancer include:

✧ anaemia
✧ fluid on the lung (pleural effusion)
✧ a tumour blocking off a large part of the lung (bronchial obstruction)
✧ a lung cancer partially blocking a lung and causing infection (collapse and consolidation)
✧ a blood clot on the lung (pulmonary embolus)
✧ the spread of cancer to other parts of the lung including the lymphatic channels (lymphangitis)

myth
Morphine is only used when no other treatments have worked and is for those who are dying.

fact
Morphine and morphine-related drugs are used at an early stage for pain control as they are one of the most effective forms of painkiller. Most people go on to have more treatment while taking morphine. People worry that they will become addicted to it but this is not the case.

✧ lung cancer occurring in lungs which have pre-existing disease (for example, chronic bronchitis or emphysema).

If it is possible to treat the underlying cause then this should be done. In cases where this has been done and breathlessness remains or where treatment is not possible then other supportive measures can be helpful. Oxygen therapy, corticosteroids and breathing exercises can be useful. Many specialist teams will offer a breathlessness service. This can be helpful in teaching people how to cope with their breathlessness by breathing exercises and energy conservation.

Cough

A cough can be troublesome. In many cases treatment of the tumour itself will help the cough but if it persists then cough suppressants and corticosteroids may be helpful.

> **my experience**
>
> My cough was very severe although I was not bringing up any phlegm. It was keeping me awake at night and I was very tired during the day. I tried most cough mixtures but they did not help. My Macmillan nurse suggested to my doctor that I try some methadone linctus at night. It seems to have worked as I can now sleep through most of the night.

Q What do Macmillan nurses do?

A Macmillan nurse can help people with cancer and their families in many ways. They can provide general advice and psychological support as well as advice on medications and symptom control.

Hoarse voice

This is usually caused by lymph glands on the left side of the mediastinum pressing on and damaging the nerve which serves the larynx

fact
Depression as a consequence of a diagnosis of lung cancer is common but often may not be diagnosed. It is important for people to discuss their feelings as well as their symptoms with the team of doctors and nurses who are looking after them. There are many effective ways of helping aspects of depression including treatment with drugs and other therapies.

or voice box. The vocal cord is paralyzed when this happens. A hoarse or weak voice can be very frustrating, especially during telephone conversations. It may be helped by referral to an ear nose and throat (ENT) surgeon who can recommend speech therapy or a small operation to the paralyzed vocal cord.

Anxiety and depression

Feelings of anxiety and depression are common when a serious illness such as lung cancer is diagnosed. People with lung cancer will feel many emotions including anger, disbelief, sadness and loss of self esteem. There is no one way of dealing with the feelings associated with being given a diagnosis of lung cancer, but discussing feelings with others can be helpful. If feelings of anxiety and depression persist then it may be reasonable for anti-depressant medication to be prescribed.

Weight loss

Weight loss is a common problem in lung cancer. Lung tumours can produce substances which affect the appetite or metabolism and cause people to lose weight rapidly – these are sometimes known as paraneoplastic syndromes (see page 36).

Treatment for lung cancer may make people feel sick, loose their sense of taste or cause difficulty in swallowing. In all of these cases dietary advice can be sought, usually from a specialist nurse or dietician.

Energy loss

Lack of energy may be a result of the cancer or the treatment for it. Many people notice that they cannot do the things they used to. Some of the problems, especially if they are related to treatment, will resolve after the treatment has been completed. If energy levels are low it can be helpful to stage activity by doing a little throughout the day rather trying to do everything at once and then feeling exhausted.

Advanced disease

Lung cancer may reach a stage where no further treatment is going to be helpful. It is particularly important that in these circumstances help and support for patients and their families is available. This can come from many sources: the specialist team at the hospital; community services; and the voluntary sector or friends and family. If possible it is better to have open discussions with all concerned, especially if a person's life expectancy is limited to days or weeks. Although possibly distressing, personal, financial or place of death arrangements may need to be discussed.

Place of death

If someone is dying of lung cancer consideration should be given as to where they wish to die. This may be at home or in a hospice or hospital. If someone wishes to die at home then usually efforts can be made to make this possible with nursing care and equipment provided as necessary.

Q What can be done to help put on weight?

A It is important to make sure that any symptoms of nausea (which can be due to the cancer or treatment) are controlled with anti-sickness medication. Eating small meals or snacks little and often may be better than sticking to main meal times. Some foods such as fresh pineapple help clear the palate and food and drinks containing ginger can help with symptoms of nausea. Occasionally drugs such as corticosteroids can be given to boost appetite.

my experience

My husband had lung cancer and after the treatment stopped working he was in a lot of pain and was admitted to the hospice who helped him with his pain. He was very anxious and when we talked he told me that he would really like to spend his last days at home but he knew I would not be able to cope on my own. I spoke to the team at the hospice and they explained to us that they could make arrangements with my GP and nurses in the community to get him home with support and help for both of us. After a few days we managed to get him home. He died a week later, quite peacefully. I cannot say that it was all plain sailing but I certainly coped with the help of the district nurses and my family. When I look back I am secure in the knowledge that he died at home where he wanted to be, surrounded by the things he was familiar with.

After death

After the death of a relative or friend with lung cancer people will experience a variety of emotions. Sometimes they will have questions about the disease or its treatment. The lung cancer team will usually be willing to try to answer these. Bereavement and support should be offered to family and friends if required and there are organizations that can help with this (see Further help section).

9

The healthcare system

Lung cancer pathway

There are many signs and symptoms of lung cancer and a diagnosis can be made in a variety of ways. If a GP suspects someone of having lung cancer they will either arrange for them to have a chest X-ray and be seen in a specialist respiratory or chest clinic or arrange for them to go directly to the chest clinic. The specialist in the chest clinic will arrange a number of tests to make a diagnosis and will usually be a member of a multi-disciplinary team (MDT). This is a group of specialists who are interested in lung cancer and who will meet regularly to discuss patients who are referred with a suspected lung cancer. Once a diagnosis has been made they will decide a plan of treatment and then discuss it with the patient and their family.

Members of the multi-disciplinary team can include:

✤ Consultant respiratory (chest) physician – a doctor who specializes in lung disease and will normally arrange the tests to make an initial diagnosis.

✤ Consultant radiologist – a doctor who performs and reports on X-rays and other imaging investigations. They may also be responsible for performing biopsies, for example, with the help of a CT scanner or ultrasound examination.

✤ Consultant pathologist – a doctor who looks at biopsies and other samples taken in order to make a diagnosis of lung cancer or not. They examine the specimens under a microscope and can do special tests on them in order to confirm a diagnosis.

✤ Consultant surgeon – a doctor who operates on lung cancer patients. There are two main types – thoracic surgeons who only operate on the lungs and associated tissues in the chest, and cardiothoracic surgeons who also operate on the heart as well as the lungs.

✤ Consultant oncologists – these doctors specialize in non-surgical treatment for lung cancer. There are two main types – clinical oncologists who give both radiotherapy and chemotherapy for lung cancer (they used to be called radiation oncologists), and medical oncologists who specialize in chemotherapy but do not give radiotherapy.

✤ Palliative care consultant – a doctor who specializes in controlling the symptoms of cancer but does not use chemotherapy or radiotherapy. They also see patients where the disease is very advanced and cannot be cured. They may have links with hospices.

✧ Other grades of doctor may attend the MDT meetings. These may include doctors in training or non-consultant grade doctors who are interested in lung cancer, for example, GPs with a special interest or staff grade doctors.

✧ Lung cancer nurse specialists – these are specially trained nurses who provide a link for patients throughout their diagnosis and treatment. They can provide both practical and psychological support and provide advice and information to patients with lung cancer and their families.

There are many others who may be part of the MDT, including:

✧ research nurses
✧ clinic nurses
✧ respiratory technicians – who perform special breathing tests
✧ radiographers – who carry out the X-ray tests
✧ physiotherapists/occupational therapists
✧ chaplaincy staff
✧ dieticians
✧ social workers
✧ Macmillan nurses
✧ clerical co-ordinators/data managers – who bring all the paperwork together.

Once a diagnosis has been made patients may see specialists in a number of different clinics or attend a joint clinic where many of the specialists in the MDT will see patients together – providing an integrated approach.

In helping to decide which treatments are best for a patient the doctor will need to assess how well the patient is able to withstand the side-effects of a particular treatment. In order to do this they will work out the performance status or score of a patient. In making this assessment they need to take into account other illnesses or medical conditions and find out how able and active a person is in their normal daily life. Research has shown that this is very accurate in predicting who benefits most from a particular treatment.

Second opinions

When someone is diagnosed with lung cancer they may have feelings of shock or disbelief. They may even question the treatment which the specialist team has proposed. It is very reasonable to ask for a full explanation as to why a particular treatment has been recommended. If genuine doubt about the proposed treatment remains then it is acceptable to ask for a second opinion of another specialist or specialist team. This can be arranged as part of the NHS although some people prefer to do this privately. In order to seek a second opinion it is usually necessary to be referred by the specialist or the GP. Most specialists will not be offended if a second opinion is requested. It is possible that in some circumstances a person is too ill or weak to seek a second opinion.

Follow up

After treatment has been completed patients should be offered follow up appropriate to their requirements.

Patients who have undergone radical or curative treatments should be offered a follow-up appointment with the specialist team to monitor the effects of treatment and to check that the cancer has not returned. Many patients who have undergone radical treatment will want to know if their treatment has been successful or not. It can be difficult to be absolutely sure as treatments such as radiotherapy carry on working after the treatment has been completed. Patients may be offered X-rays to monitor their response to treatment.

Patients who have undergone palliative treatment should be offered a personal follow-up plan that best fits their needs. This may take the form of follow-up appointments at the hospital, possibly in a nurse-led clinic, or back in the community with their GP. Access back to the specialist service can be made if their GP or other healthcare workers in the community feel that it may be helpful.

Q **Do I need a scan when my treatment has been completed?**

A Whether a scan is needed or not depends on the aim of the treatment. If the treatment is to cure the lung cancer then a scan may help in deciding whether all the cancer has gone. Scans can only detect cancer above a certain size so they are not foolproof. If the aim of treatment is palliative and to help symptoms then the most important aspect of the treatment is whether those symptoms are better and a scan is not essential. If a patient is taking part in a clinical trial, then more information about the treatment being tested will be required and extra scans may be needed.

Hospices

Hospices can provide valuable support and treatment for lung cancer patients. In the past many people felt that hospices were places where people with terminal illnesses went to die. Although hospices can provide care for people who are terminally ill they also provide many more services. These include:

✧ rehabilitation after cancer treatment
✧ respite care
✧ out-patient clinics for symptom control
✧ in-patient stay for symptom control
✧ day-care facilities
✧ complementary therapies
✧ psychological and bereavement support.

myth
Hospices are places to go to die.

fact
Hospices have many functions. They provide help with controlling symptoms, rehabilitation after cancer treatment and support for families and carers. Many people are discharged home after being in a hospice.

my experience
When my lung cancer had spread to my bones I was in a lot of pain and my doctor and Macmillan nurse had difficulty in finding the correct medication to control the pain. They suggested that I came into the local hospice. I was very reluctant as I felt that if I went in there I would never come out alive. In the hospice the doctors and nurses could monitor my pain closely and assess the changes they made to my medication. I also had a nerve block performed which helped my pain considerably. The atmosphere was not gloomy and I found it much more relaxing than being in a hospital ward. If I have to go into the hospice again I won't be afraid.

Community support

Although a lot of the diagnosis and treatment of lung cancer will take place in hospital there is a lot of helpful information and support available in the community. GPs provide continuity and basic medical advice. District nurses provide nursing care and support, usually in a patient's own home. Macmilllan nurses can provide information and support for patients and their families for all stages of lung cancer. Marie Curie Nurses can provide home nursing care for lung cancer patients when the disease is in the terminal stages.

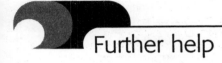 Further help

The British Lung Foundation (BLF)

The British Lung Foundation is the only UK-based charity dedicated to helping and supporting people with all lung diseases through provision of comprehensive and clear information on paper, on the web, on the telephone and by running a nationwide network of Breathe Easy support groups. The BLF also works for positive change in lung health. They do this by campaigning, raising awareness and funding world-class research.

British Lung Foundation
73–5 Goswell Road
London EC1V 7ER

Helpline (staffed by specialist respiratory nurses and benefits advisers): 08458 505020
www.lunguk.org

CancerBACKUP (formally known as CancerBACUP)

CancerBACKUP was launched as a national cancer information service in 1985. It provides high quality and up-to-date information, practical advice and support with a free cancer information service staffed by qualified and experienced cancer nurses. It also produces publications on all aspects of cancer written specifically for patients and their families.

CancerBACKUP
3 Bath Place
Rivington Street
London EC2A 3JR
Tel: 020 7696 9003
(Switchboard open during
office hours, Mon–Fri,
9:00 a.m–5:30 p.m.)
Fax: 020 7696 9002
Cancer information helpline
(UK only):
0808 800 1234 (freephone)
020 7739 2280 (standard rate)
(Lines are staffed by cancer
specialist nurses, Mon–Fri,
9:00 a.m–8:00 p.m.)
www.cancerbackup.org.uk

CancerHelp UK

CancerHelp UK is a free information
service about cancer and cancer
care for people with cancer and
their families. It is provided by
Cancer Research UK. It believes that
information about cancer should be
freely available to all and its
literature is written in a way that
people can easily understand.

Cancer Information Department
Cancer Research UK
PO Box 123
Lincoln's Inn Fields
London WC2A 3PX

Tel: 020 7061 8355
    0800 226 237
www.cancerhelp.org.uk

Cancerlink

Cancerlink helps people with cancer
and helps their friends and families
to live with cancer. It provides
information, emotional support and
practical advice.

11–21 Northdown Street
London N1 9BN
Tel: 0808 808 2020
www.cancerlink.org.uk

Cancer Research UK

Cancer Research UK is the UK's
leading charity dedicated to cancer
research. The Cancer Research UK
website contains a large amount of
information about cancer.

Cancer Research UK
PO Box 123
Lincoln's Inn Fields
London WC2A 3PX
Tel: 020 7121 6699
(Supporter services)
Tel: 020 7242 0200
(Switchboard)
Fax: 020 7269 3100
www.cancerresearchuk.org

CRUSE Bereavement Care

CRUSE Bereavement Care exists to promote the wellbeing of bereaved people and to enable anyone bereaved to understand their grief and cope with their loss. The organization provides counselling and support. It offers information, advice, education and training services.

Tel: 0844 477 9400
Young person's freephone helpline:
0808 808 1677
email: helpline@cruse.org.uk

Macmillan Cancer Relief

Macmillan Cancer Relief is a UK charity that works to improve the quality of life for people living with cancer. Macmillan offers life support by providing the expert care and practical support that makes a real difference to people living with cancer. They offer a range of innovative cancer services through-out the UK.

Macmillan Cancer Relief
Anchor House
15–19 Britten Street
London SW3 3TZ
Tel: 020 7840 7840

Macmillan CancerLine

For information or emotional support for patients and their families contact the Macmillan CancerLine:

Freephone: 0808 808 2020
(Mon–Fri, 9:00 a.m.–6:00 p.m.)
e-mail: cancerline@
macmillan.org.uk
www.macmillan.org.uk

Maggie's Centres

Maggie's Centres is a charitable organization for anybody who has or has had, cancer. It is also for their families, their friends and their carers. It provides centres close to a major cancer hospital treatment centre in order to allow people to take time out and to give them a non-institutional place that they can call their own.

There are now Maggie's Centres in Edinburgh, Glasgow, Dundee, Inverness and Oxford. Further centres are planned in a number of other towns. Details of all the centres and contact details can be obtained by visiting their website: www.maggiescentres.org.

Marie Curie Cancer Care

Marie Curie Cancer Care is a charitable organization that provides care to cancer patients and their families. It provides community nursing care for terminally ill people and has ten hospices around the UK for care of patients and support of their carers. Referral to a hospice is usually arranged by a GP or a hospital doctor. The Marie Curie Research Institute aides research in the investigation of the causes and better ways to treat the disease.

England (head office)
Marie Curie Cancer Care
89 Albert Embankment
London SE1 7TP
Tel: 020 7599 7777
Scotland
29 Albany Street
Edinburgh EH1 3QN
Tel: 0131 456 3700

Wales
Raglan Chambers
63 Frogmore Street
Abergavenny
Monmouthshire NP7 5AN
Tel: 01873 30 3000

Northern Ireland
60 Knock Road
Belfast BT5 6LQ
Tel: 028 9088 2060

QUIT

QUIT is an independent charity whose aim is to save lives by helping smokers to stop.

QUIT
Ground Floor
211 Old Street
London EC1V 9NR
Tel: 020 7251 1551
Fax: 020 7251 1661
email: info@quit.org.uk
Free help quit line: 0800 00 22 00
www.quit.org.uk

Roy Castle Lung Cancer Foundation

The Roy Castle Lung Cancer Foundation is the only charity in the UK dedicated to defeating lung cancer through research, campaigning and education. It also provides practical and emotional support for patients and all those affected by lung cancer and smoking.

The Roy Castle Lung Cancer
Foundation
200 London Road, Liverpool
Merseyside L3 9TA
Tel: 0871 220 5426
Fax: 0871 220 5427
www.roycastle.org

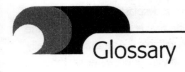

Glossary

abdominal cavity
The cavity that holds the stomach, liver, gall bladder, spleen, pancreas, urinary bladder and intestines.

acute side-effects
Side-effects which occur during or immediately after treatment.

adjuvant
Treatment which is given in addition to the main treatment.

adrenal glands
Glands which sit adjacent to the top of the kidneys and produce steroids and adrenaline.

alveoli
The minute air sacs found at the end of the bronchial tubes. There are several million in each lung and it is through these that oxygen passes into the bloodstream and carbon dioxide passes out of the bloodstream.

asbestos related lung disease
Asbestos can cause a number of conditions that affect the lung or the lining of the lung including benign pleural plaques, asbestosis and malignant mesothelioma.

benign
A non-cancerous tumour.

biopsy
The removal of a small piece of tissue in order to make a diagnosis.

bone marrow	Blood-making cells situated in bones.
cancer protecting gene	A protective gene that normally limits the growth of tumours. Also known as a tumour suppressor gene. If such a gene is mutated it may fail to stop a cancer from developing.
cannula	A thin, hollow tube used to introduce fluid (or medication) to, or remove it from, the body.
carcinogen	A cancer promoting agent.
carcinoid syndrome	The symptoms of carcinoid syndrome commonly include flushing, diarrhoea, abdominal pain and wheezing.
carcinoma-in-situ	Meaning 'cancer-in-place', represents the final transformation of a dysplastic cell to cancer.
chest drain	A soft plastic tube that is inserted between the ribs into the pleural space. The drain is usually attached to a one-way underwater seal that allows air or fluid out of the pleural space but does not allow it back in again.
chronic bronchitis	Chronic inflammation of the airways caused by cigarette smoke.
co-morbidities	Other illnesses or conditions that a patient with lung cancer might have.
consultant respiratory physician	A hospital-based doctor who specializes in lung diseases. Sometimes referred to as a chest physician or lung specialist.
contrast	A special injection of dye given just before a CT scan that outlines the blood vessels and helps the radiologist to identify the blood vessels in the chest.
coronary angiography	An X-ray picture of the blood vessels that supply the heart muscle. A fine, hollow tube called a catheter is introduced into an artery in the forearm or groin and is advanced through the blood vessels until the heart is reached. A dye is then injected into the blood vessels and X-rays taken from several angles. This allows a 'road map' of the blood vessels supplying the heart

	muscle to be drawn, showing where they are narrowed and how narrow they have become.
creatinine	A natural by-product of metabolism that is excreted by the kidneys.
CT scan	Computed tomography scan.
cytotoxic drugs	Drugs used as part of chemotherapy to kill cancer cells.
deep vein thrombosis (DVT)	A blood clot that can develop in one of the large veins inside the leg or pelvis.
dysplastic epithelium	Abnormal change in the lining of the airway. Although such changes can sometimes regress spontaneously, dysplasia is believed to be a pre-cancerous change.
echocardiogram	An ultrasound test to look at the heart and the tissues surrounding it.
emphysema	Irreversible destruction of lung tissue caused by cigarette smoke.
empyema	Pus in the pleural space around the lung.
endobronchial treatments	Techniques used to treat tumours that are positioned inside the airways.
enzymes	Proteins which help biological reactions take place.
epidemiology	The study of patterns of disease.
erythropoietin	A naturally occurring protein which stimulates bone marrow to make red blood cells. It can be given as a drug by injection under the skin to help treat anaemia related to chemotherapy.
fibrosis	Lung fibrosis involves scarring of the lung. Gradually, the air sacs of the lungs become replaced by fibrotic tissue. When the scar forms, the tissue becomes thicker causing an irreversible loss of the tissue's ability to transfer oxygen into the bloodstream. In some cases no cause can be identified – this is called idiopathic lung fibrosis.
fistula	Abnormal connection between two parts of the body.

fraction	The term given to a single radiotherapy treatment.
frozen section	A biopsy which is frozen immediately after removal and examined by a pathologist during the operation.
GCSF	A naturally occurring protein which can be given as a drug by injection to stimulate the production of white cells.
gene	Sequence of DNA required to produce a protein.
GFR	Glomerular Filtration Rate. A measurement of how well the kidneys are working.
glucose	A type of sugar.
gray	A Gray (Gy) is a unit of radiation dose.
growth factors	Substances which circulate in the body and have an effect on cells, usually by attaching to receptors and causing cells to become more active.
haemoglobin	An iron-containing protein which carries oxygen around the body to tissues.
haemoptysis	A condition where the patient coughs up blood or sputum containing blood.
hilum	The root of the lungs where the lobar bronchi join the main bronchi.
Hodgkin's disease	A type of lymphoma – cancer of the lymph glands.
hypercalcaemia	Elevated calcium levels in the blood.
incidence	The number of new cases of a disease occurring per year.
intravenous	A drug given directly into a vein via a small sterile tube or cannula.
intravenous injection	Injection into a vein.
jaundice	Yellow discolouration of the skin and the whites of the eyes due to deposition of bile pigments in the tissues.
linear accelerator	A machine that is capable of delivering high energy X-rays to treat cancer.
lobar bronchi	A bronchus that supplies one lobe of the lung.

lobe	Segment of the lung.
lobectomy	The removal of a single lobe of the lung, together with the lymph glands at the root of the lung.
lymph nodes	Small, bean-shaped structures scattered along vessels of the lymphatic system. These glands act as filters collecting bacteria and cancer cells that may travel through the lymphatic system.
lymphatic vessels	Vessels that carry lymph fluid to and from the lymph glands.
main bronchus	An airway that supplies air to one lung.
magnesium and potassium salts	Chemicals which occur naturally in the body and which are essential for metabolism.
malignant	A tumour that is able to spread and grow in other parts of the body.
mediastinum	The area between the lungs that contains the heart, major blood vessels and windpipe.
medical physicist	A scientist specially trained in the use of radiation to treat tumours.
metastasis	The spread of a disease, especially cancer, from one part of the body to another via the bloodstream or lymphatic system.
metastasize	The ability of a cancer to spread to other parts of the body to form secondary cancers (metastases). Lung cancers commonly spread to the liver, brain, bones, other lung and adrenal glands in the abdomen.
Metformin	Tablet medication given to some people who have diabetes.
micro-metastatic disease	Disease which has spread in an amount so small it cannot be seen by conventional scans or blood tests.
monoclonal antibodies	Special proteins which recognize a particular receptor on a cell surface.
mutation	Alteration in the DNA sequence of a cell.
multi-disciplinary meeting	A group of specialists interested in lung cancer who meet regularly to discuss patients who

are referred with lung cancer or suspected lung cancer. They decide on the best use of tests to make a diagnosis and advise on treatment.

neuroendocrine tumours
There are several types of neuroendocrine lung tumours which arise from specialized cells in the lung called neuroendocrine cells. The most serious type is small cell lung cancer. The other two main types of neuroendocrine tumours are typical and atypical carcinoids.

neurosurgery
Surgery on the brain or spinal cord.

neutrophils
A type of white blood cell which help the body fight infection. (Also known as granulocytes.)

NSCLC
Non-small cell lung cancer.

nucleus
The control centre of a cell.

oncogene
Tumour gene present in the body that can be activated and cause cells to grow and divide in an uncontrolled manner.

oncology
The area of medicine that deals with the study and the treatment of cancer.

palliative treatment
A treatment which is not designed to cure but to help alleviate or prevent symptoms.

pancoast tumour
A lung cancer that develops at the apex of the lung and invades nearby tissues, such as the ribs and vertebrae.

paraneoplastic syndromes
The collective signs and symptoms caused by a substance produced from a tumour or in reaction to a tumour.

paraplegia
Weakness and sometimes loss of power of both legs caused by damage to the spinal cord.

performance status
A simple 0–4 scale that describes everyday activities that a patient with cancer is capable of undertaking and their ability to have treatment.

pericardiocentesis
Drainage of a pericardial effusion.

pericardial sac
A sac of thin tissues which contains the heart.

photoactive drug
A drug that is activated by light.

pleura	Membrane lining the lung (visceral pleura) and the inside of the rib cage (parietal pleura).
pleural effusion	Fluid that accumulates between the pleural membranes.
pneumonectomy	The removal of an entire lung along with the associated lymph glands.
pneumothorax	Air in the pleural space.
prevalence	A measure of how common a condition or activity is, at any one time.
prognosis	Forecast of the probable or expected outcome of a disease.
radical treatment	A treatment aimed at curing the cancer.
radiographer	An individual trained to plan and administer radiation therapy.
radiation oncologist	A doctor who specializes in radiation therapy to cancers. Sometimes known in the UK as a clinical oncologist.
receptor	A protein on the surface of a cell which acts as a switch for activities within the cell.
risk factor	Anything that increases your chance of getting a disease.
saline solution	Salt water.
SCLC	Small cell lung cancer.
segmentectomy	The removal of a segment of a lobe. Each lobe of the lung is composed of several segments.
simulator	A machine which mimics the linear accelerator but takes diagnostic X-rays so that the details can be checked before starting treatment on the linear accelerator.
sleeve resection	The removal of the upper or middle lobe and affected area of bronchus. The healthy lower lobe is then re-implanted onto remaining healthy bronchus.
specialist cancer nurse	An experienced nurse who specializes in the care of patients with cancer.
stent	An expandable hollow tube.

stereotactic radiotherapy/ gamma knife radiosurgery
A type of highly focused radiotherapy where the radiation beams are directed at a small tumour deposit.

stridor
A high pitched, harsh noise caused by partial airway obstruction.

thoracotomy
A surgical procedure to open up the chest.

thorax
Area inside the ribs where the lungs and heart are situated.

tinnitus
Ringing in the ears.

trachea
Also known as the windpipe. An air tube, usually stiffened by rings of cartilage, that extends from the voicebox to the bronchus of each lung.

wedge resection
The removal of a small wedge-shaped portion of lung.

wheeze
A continuous, coarse, whistling sound produced during breathing.

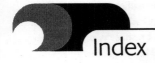

Index

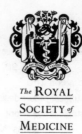

The ROYAL
SOCIETY of
MEDICINE

The Royal Society of Medicine (RSM) is an independent medical charity with a primary aim to provide continuing professional development for qualified medical and health-related professionals. The public benefits from health care professionals who have received high quality and relevant education from the RSM.

The Society celebrated its bicentenary in 2005. Each year it arranges and holds over 400 meetings for health care professionals across a wide range of medical subjects. In order to aid education and further training the Society also has the largest postgraduate medical library in Europe – based in central London together with online access to specialist databases. RSM Press, the Society's publishing arm, publishes books and journals principally aimed at the medical profession.

A number of conferences and events are held each year for the public as well as members of the Society. These include the successful 'Medicine and Me' series, designed to bring together patients, their carers and the medical profession. In addition, the RSM's Open and History of Medicine Sections arrange meetings on a regular basis which can be attended by the public.

In addition to the lectures and training provided by the RSM, members of the Society also have access to club facilities including accommodation and a restaurant. The conference and meeting facilities of the RSM were refurbished for their bicentenary and are available to the public for hire for meetings and seminars. In addition, Chandos House, a beautifully restored Georgian townhouse, designed by Robert Adam, is also now available to hire for training, receptions and weddings (as it has a civil wedding licence).

To find out more about the Royal Society of Medicine and the work it undertakes please visit www.rsm.ac.uk or call 020 7290 2991. For more information about RSM Press, please visit www.rsmpress.co.uk.